KETO APPETIZER COOKBOOK

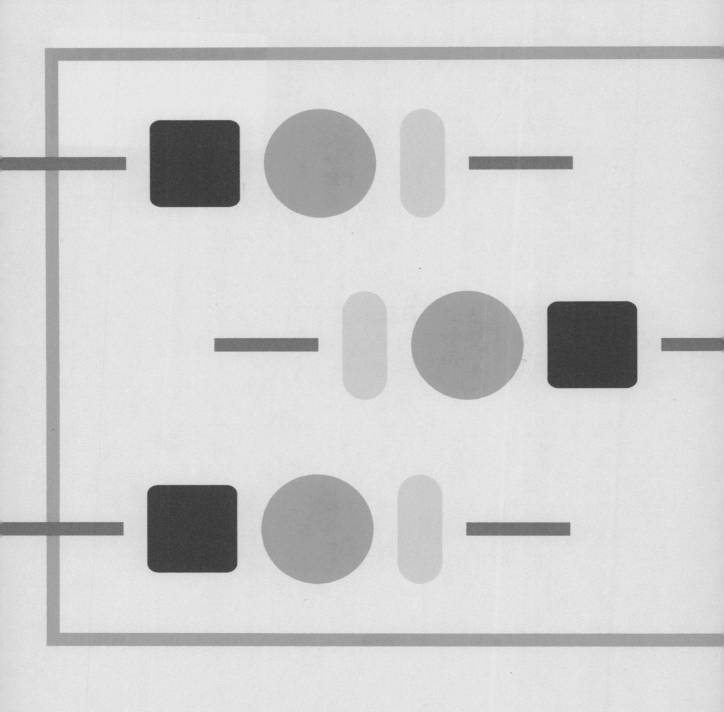

Keto Appetizer
COOKBOOK

60 Delicious Low-Carb Favorites

DAMILOLA
APATA

ROCKRIDGE
PRESS

First Rockridge Press trade paperback edition 2022

Rockridge Press and the Rockridge Press logo are trademarks or registered trademarks of Callisto Media Inc. and/or its affiliates in the United States and other countries and may not be used without written permission.

For general information on our other products and services, please contact our Customer Care Department within the United States at (866) 744-2665, or outside the United States at (510) 253-0500.

Some of the recipes originally appeared, in different form, in *Ketogenic Diet on a Budget: Shop Smarter, Batch Cook, and Eat Better*; *Super Easy Keto Cookbook: 100 Simple Ketogenic Diet Recipes*; *The Pescatarian Keto Cookbook: 100 Recipes and a 14-Day Meal Plan to Burn Fat and Boost Health*; *Keto Comfort Food Classics: Your Favorite Recipes Made Keto*; *7-Day Keto: The Starter Guide for Ketogenic Diet Beginners*; *She Does Keto: The Complete Ketogenic Diet for Women*; *The Southern Keto Cookbook: 100 High-Fat, Low-Carb Recipes for Classic Comfort Food*; *Essential Ketogenic Mediterranean Diet Cookbook: 100 Low-Carb, Heart-Healthy Recipes for Lasting Weight Loss*; *Keto for Vegetarians: Lose Weight and Improve Health on a Plant-Based Ketogenic Diet*; and *Anti-Inflammatory Keto Cookbook: 100 Recipes and a 2-Week Plan to Jump-Start Your Healing*.

Paperback ISBN: 978-1-63878-417-3
eBook ISBN: 978-1-63878-980-2

Manufactured in the United States of America

Interior and Cover Designer: Scott A. Woodledge
Art Producer: Sue Bischofberger
Editor: Leah Zarra
Production Editor: Rachel Taenzler
Production Manager: Jose Olivera

Photography © Laura Flippen, cover and p. 67; © Evi Abeler, pp. vi-vii and 61; © from_my_point_of_view/iStock.com, p. x; © Darren Muir, p. 8; © Andrew Purcell, pp. 14 and 17; © Hélène Dujardin, p. 23; © vaaseenaa/iStock, p. 27; © AlexPro9500/iStock, pp. 42 and 87; © Emulsion Studio, p. 64; © Nadine Greeff, pp. 94 and 115; and © Shea Evans, p. 105. Author photo courtesy of Tiffany Couture Photography.
Cover image: Caprese-Stuffed Avocados (page 37)

10 9 8 7 6 5 4 3 2 1 0

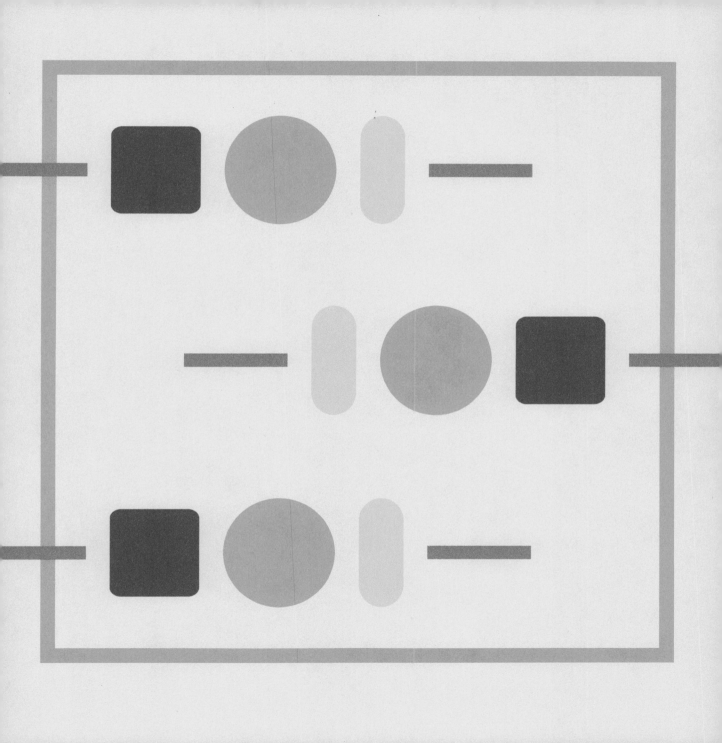

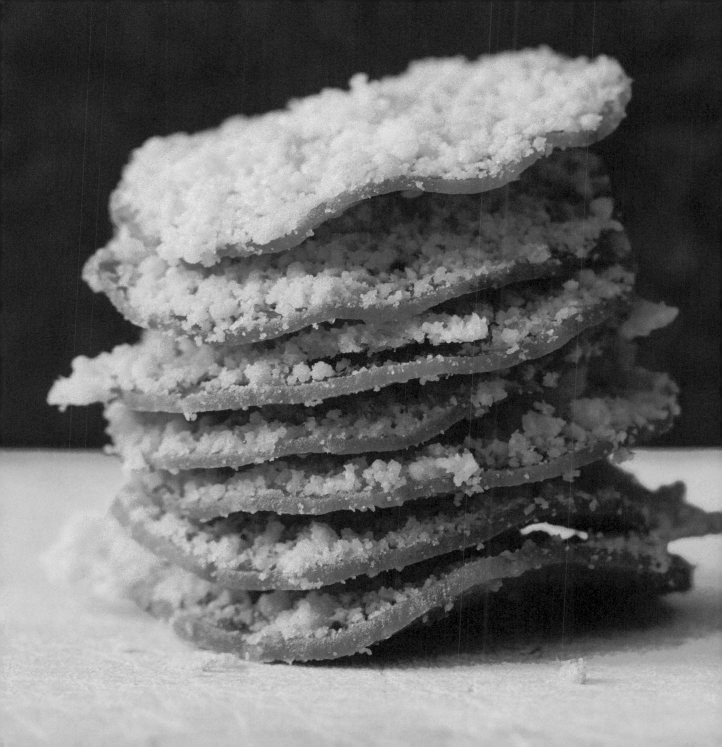

Contents

◀ Pepperoni-Parmesan Chips (page 83)

Introduction

I am absolutely a believer in the keto diet and all its benefits. I was introduced to the keto lifestyle in 2017 and have followed it on and off, primarily for weight loss, for the last five years. I had tried almost every single diet you can think of—all of them were short-lived and proved unsustainable for me. There were so many "off-limits" foods and no replacements to fill that void. I love that the keto diet offers a wide variety of foods you can enjoy without feeling deprived.

If you're like me, you might like to host a nice get-together every once in a while. Whether it's a potluck, a gameday party, or simply a movie night with friends, you're always down for the cause. What goes hand-in-hand with entertaining? Food, of course! Fun, festive appetizers are often the highlight of any event. Would you like to be able to host a party and keep your nutritional goals intact? Have you been assigned to bring a dish and would like to keep it keto friendly? If so, this book is for you. You shouldn't have to give up your favorite dishes to adapt to a keto lifestyle. Instead, try using keto-friendly substitutes to re-create your favorite snacks and appetizers. Having the option to re-create so many meals in a keto-friendly manner is one of the main reasons for my success with this diet.

The recipes in this book will all be keto compliant so you don't have to worry about being kicked out of ketosis. You'll find 60 delicious recipes that you'll end up making time and time again. Your guests won't even know that the delicious appetizers they're enjoying are keto friendly!

In this book, you'll find nuggets of information, like the best keto substitutes for common ingredients and tips and tricks for how to make the best version of each dish listed. The recipes also touch on different types of cuisines and cultures. You can expand your flavor palate, all while remaining in ketosis. Furthermore, there's a nice variety of savory and sweet recipes for your liking. Nothing brings guests together like appetizers, and the recipes in this book are sure to wow them. You may even get a few keto converts as a result of the delicious food you'll be offering! You're bound to have multiple people asking you for the recipes at the end of the day.

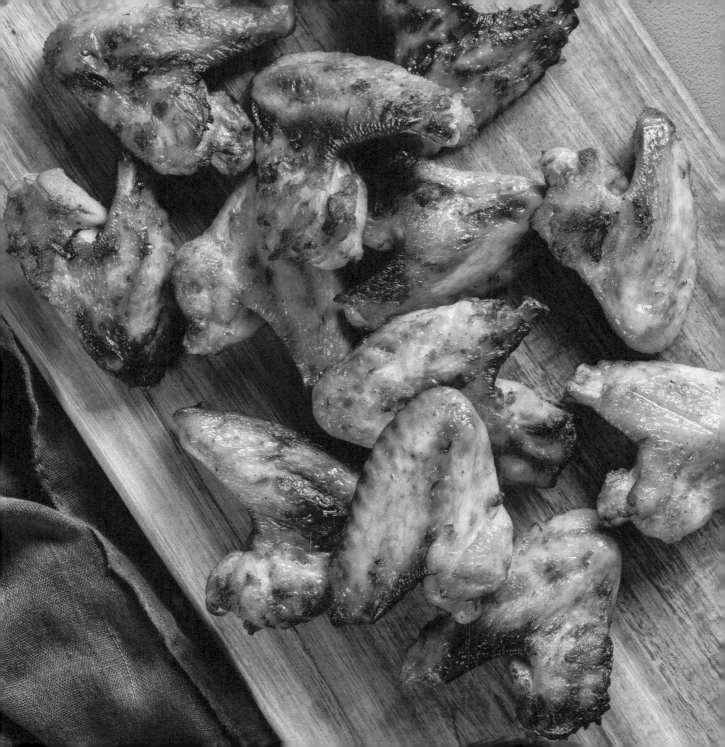

CHAPTER 1

Welcome Appetizers to the Keto Party

Transforming your favorite appetizers to fit your keto lifestyle should not be a challenge or a struggle. Everyone loves a good selection of appetizers at a party, and keto appetizers are not any different. Our main goal is to keep the fats high and the carbs low, so the possibilities are endless. You do not have to fill up your plate with only celery, carrots, and cheese while others enjoy a wide selection of snacks and apps. Whether you're hosting a fancy dinner or a gameday watch party, you'll surely find keto-friendly appetizer recipes to fit any and every event.

◀ Sriracha Wings (page 20)

Apps-solutely Keto

It seems like everywhere you turn, there's a new keto book out. A lot of these books focus on creating breakfast, lunch, and dinner options. A few even hone in on how to master keto desserts and meal prep. However, the world of keto appetizers has yet to be thoroughly explored. You can never have too many appetizers. They're designed to stimulate your taste buds and prepare you for the meal ahead, though they often end up being the star of the show. Satiation, being full, is one of the main objectives of the keto diet, so curating appetizers that are filled with plenty of healthy fats and proteins falls right in line with your goals. Appetizers also often double as snacks, so if you have leftovers from an event, you can incorporate them into the next day's meal plan and keep the party going.

Whether this is your first attempt at the keto diet or counting carbs is practically second nature to you, you'll find yourself wanting a snack or appetizer every now and then. As long as you are remaining within your macros and making a conscious effort to keep your carbs minimal, you have no problem. Are you planning an event and in need of various keto-friendly options? Were you invited to a potluck, and now you're confused on what to bring in order to stay on track? Do you simply love to snack and graze on any given day? Regardless of which category you fall into, you'll find something in this book for you!

Keto Refresher

No matter your keto experience thus far—whether you're a master of macros or this is your first time trying out the diet—this book will certainly prove helpful. Let's go through a quick little keto refresher, shall we? What is the ketogenic diet? The simple answer is that it's a low-carb, high-fat, and moderate protein diet. The goal of the ketogenic diet is to reduce your carbohydrate intake to the point where your body converts to burning fat as its primary source of fuel. Carbohydrates come in different forms, such as sugars, starches, and fibers. Most people automatically think of bread, pasta, potatoes, and rice when it comes to carbs; however, we must keep in mind that some fruits and vegetables, such as pineapples, mangos, and corn, also contain high amounts of carbohydrates. Various sodas, juices, and cocktails also rank high in carbs due to their high sugar content. It is important to keep an eye out for the types of foods and ingredients that contain a lot of carbs so you can be sure to limit or avoid them and remain in ketosis. Once you get the hang of how to properly eat on keto, you can begin to reap all of its benefits, too.

Mind Your Macros

The nutrients we use in the highest amounts—fat, protein, and carbohydrates—are called macronutrients, also known as macros. Your main focus when on keto is to build your meals primarily of healthy fats, followed by proteins. In order to follow a ketogenic diet, simply look at your caloric intake and construct it as follows:

Fat: 70–80%	Protein: 10–20%	Carbohydrates: 5–10%

For some, the amount allocated to carbs seems extremely small. The good news is most people count "net carbs" instead of total carbs. Net carbs are calculated by subtracting dietary fiber and sugar alcohols from total carbohydrates—the dietary fiber and sugar alcohols are discounted because the body cannot digest them. This gives you a wider variety of foods to consume because, although the total carbs on an item may be higher, the net carbs may still fit within your macros.

Now, different people on the keto diet will follow different ratios. Some may follow a higher-protein-style diet due to intense workouts or simply pure preference. Others may choose to reduce their protein intake to as little as possible, maximizing the increased energy from fat. One thing that stays consistent throughout different versions of keto is the lack of carbs. The most keto-friendly ingredients consist mainly of fats and proteins. Look at cream cheese, for example: Two tablespoons of cream cheese contain roughly 9 grams of total fat, 2 grams of carbohydrates, and 2 grams of protein. As you can see, the category with the highest percentage is fat. Cream cheese makes for an excellent addition to so many appetizers (see Jalapeño Firecrackers, page 50), so it's ideal that it has macros that align with your keto goals.

Keeping Up with Ketosis

As mentioned earlier, ketosis is a metabolic state whereby your body is using fat as its energy source instead of carbohydrates. Normally, your body would be converting carbohydrates to energy, but since you've nearly eliminated your carb intake, your body has no choice but to find an alternative way to function. Following a ketogenic diet has been shown to have many great benefits, such as increased energy levels, reduced high blood pressure, and even improved insulin sensitivity.

Recently, the keto diet has become popular for its most common benefit, weight loss. Why is weight loss so common on the keto diet? Well, if your body has naturally switched over into consistently burning fat to use as an energy source, you're pretty much a walking, talking, fat-burning machine! As the fat melts away, you'll begin to not only notice a change in your body composition but also a lower number on the scale. Some followers of the ketogenic diet also reported a reversal of their type 2 diabetes.

There are different ways to track whether or not you're in ketosis. The most common ways are by testing the ketones in your blood using a urinalysis ketone strip or using a blood glucose and ketone reader to measure the ketones in your blood. Unfortunately, life throws curveballs at you, and you may have times where you've kicked yourself out of ketosis. The best thing to do is to drink lots of water and immediately cut out carbs and return to the keto diet. You'll be back on track and burning fat in no time!

Naturally Keto App Staples

The appetizers in this book will be the talk of the party, and luckily most of them incorporate foods that are already keto staples. Take a look at some of the ingredients you'll find in many of these recipes:

Almond flour: You'll find this baked into various keto breads and crackers. It's important to make sure you're getting almond flour and not almond meal, which is not as finely milled and can yield dramatically different results.

Cream cheese: This will be the base of different fat bombs and the foundation of multiple dips. If your recipe calls for many other high-fat ingredients, you can balance them out by choosing a reduced-fat cream cheese, if you want slightly lower calories.

Parmesan cheese: This salty ingredient stars as way more than a topping in several recipes. It makes for the perfect breading and can stand alone to form the crispiest crackers (see Crispy Parmesan Crackers, page 92). I suggest using powdered or grated Parmesan cheese for breading because it has the texture most similar to flour. If you want to make a recipe vegetarian, make sure to buy vegetarian-friendly Parmesan, as most Parmesan is made using animal rennet or enzymes.

Eggs: Aside from a delicious deviled egg recipe (page 22), eggs can be found in almost every baked recipe in this book. Be sure to take your eggs out of the refrigerator so they can be room temperature by the time you're starting your recipe.

Olive oil: This pure fat is light tasting and featured as a drizzle over some keto-friendly finger foods and as a binder in various bread recipes. I prefer to use extra-virgin olive oil, since it has the best taste.

Keto-Friendly Drinks

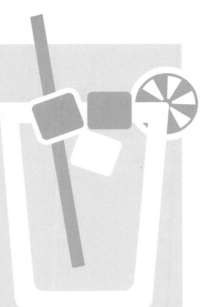

Drinking tends to be an integral part of parties and social gatherings. The great thing about the keto diet is that you do not have to omit alcohol or stick to water at every occasion. Most pure spirits such as rum, vodka, gin, tequila, and whiskey do not contain any carbohydrates at all. What you need to be mindful of is the mixers you use to form your crafty cocktails. One wrong addition can quickly turn your keto-friendly cocktail into a sugar-loaded surprise. Opt to mix your alcohols with diet sodas or zero-sugar juices. Some people even prefer to spice up their drinks using sugar-free powdered flavor packets or liquid water enhancers. Don't be fooled by tonic water, either! Did you know that just one can of regular tonic water contains 32 grams of sugar? To keep your carbs low, opt for diet tonic water instead!

If hard liquor isn't quite your vibe, there are alternatives for you as well. Many companies have created light beers and sugar-free seltzers to help you stay on track with your fitness goals. Although these items may not be zero carbs, almost all of them come in fewer than 4 net carbs. Champagne, red wine, and white wine are also drinks you can enjoy. The key is to stay away from the sweeter wines like moscato. Instead, you should opt for dry wines to keep your carb count low. And of course, if alcohol isn't for you, feel free to stick to the diet sodas and zero-sugar juices for enjoyment.

Easy Keto Swaps

If you're worried that some of your favorite appetizers can't be transformed into keto-friendly snacks, you've come to the right place! Sometimes all it takes is a few ingredient swaps here and there in order to keep your dish in alignment with keto standards. You'd be surprised at just how many different recipes you can re-create and enjoy when on keto. As with any keto dish, proteins are always permitted, so if Buffalo wings, shrimp cocktail, or barbecue meatballs are your appetizers of choice, you definitely won't be missing out on anything! Dips and sauces are also easy to throw together and often will not require too many adjustments.

The key things to look out for are high-carb items. Foods that usually accompany dips, like chips, crackers, and toast, are the ingredients you'll want to swap out. You'll also want to keep an eye out for any sweet sauces or glazes. The sugar content can sneak up on you easily, so make sure to incorporate your favorite keto-friendly sweetener in place of regular sugar! Take a look at the following chart for a few examples of some of the keto-friendly swaps you can use to adjust your favorite recipes.

INGREDIENT	SWAP(S)
Breadcrumbs	Crushed pork rinds, Parmesan cheese, crushed nuts
Sugar	Stevia, erythritol, xylitol, monk fruit, allulose
Chips	Pork rinds, halved mini bell peppers, sliced cucumber or radishes, pepperoni crisps
Crackers	Cheese crisps, almond-flour crackers, flaxseed crackers
Flour	Almond flour, coconut flour, lupin flour

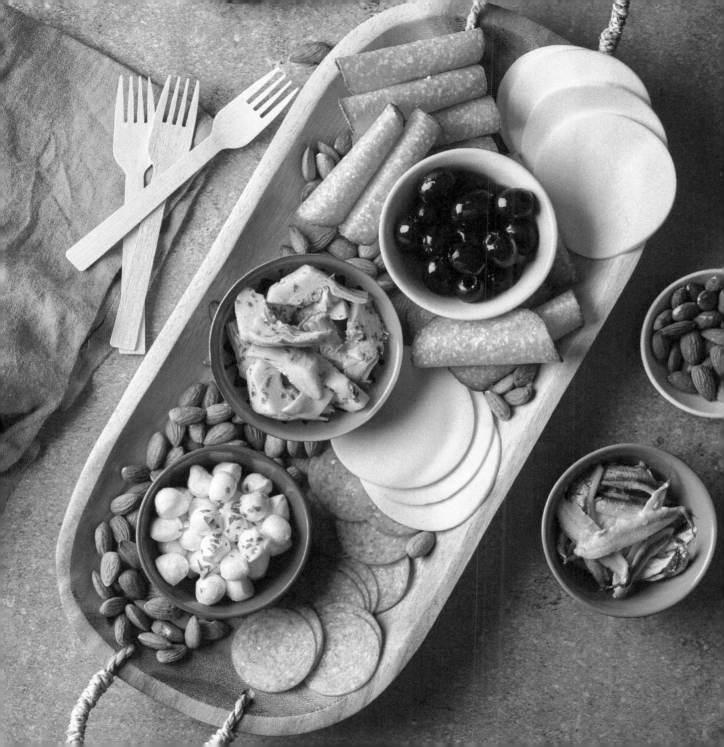

Assembling Charcuterie Plates

Charcuterie boards are an artistic way to add plenty of keto options to your appetizer lineup. They often consist of a variety of meats and cheeses as the base, with a few other additions such as fruits, vegetables, nuts, and crackers to fill up the space. I love charcuterie boards because they allow each guest to curate their own plate tailored to their individual tastes. Since meats and cheeses are the base of keto, feel free to pile them onto your board.

My favorite meats to use are various salami because you can get a nice, perfectly round cut. For cheeses, the options are endless. I like to use a mix of soft and hard cheeses so my guests have plenty to choose from. Brie is my soft cheese of choice for its slightly buttery taste. As for hard cheeses, my go-to is classic cheddar because it pairs well with so many things. Remember, you're not limited to just meat and cheese. Consider adding fresh berries, cucumbers, pickles, and low-carb nuts such as almonds, pecans, and macadamia nuts to spice up your board. I like a variety of colors on charcuterie boards, so I try placing the different items based on their colors. You can create paper tent labels by folding small pieces of paper and placing them around the charcuterie board to let guests know what each item is. You can have fun and get creative with your board, all while keeping it keto friendly.

Planning and Prep Tips

It's simple to plan and host events for both keto and non-keto guests. Many every-day ingredients can be put together to make a keto-friendly appetizer. Consider the following tips when preparing the recipes in this book and planning a party for a variety of guests:

1. **Pick dishes that everyone can enjoy regardless of a "label."** When you hear Maple Bacon-Wrapped Brussels Sprouts (page 30), your mind does not automatically think keto—because this recipe uses common ingredients enjoyed by all.

2. **Make your dips and spreads the day before.** I find that most dips and spreads taste better the following day after all the flavors have had a chance to meld together. Preparing them ahead will also save you some time for more time-consuming dishes.

3. **Arrange non-keto ingredients together.** To be mindful of your guests who do follow the keto diet, you can put high-carb items together so they aren't mis-taken for a keto replacement. The last thing you want is for someone in ketosis to devour crackers made with white flour instead of almond flour.

4. **Purchase presliced meats and cheeses for charcuterie boards.** You may not want to spend all your time slicing salami or chopping cheddar. Most grocery stores sell a variety of meats and cheeses presliced into all shapes and sizes for your convenience.

5. **Encourage your non-keto guests to try the keto-friendly appetizers.** You'd be surprised at how much of a hit these appetizers will be. The more guests you have that can enjoy your keto dishes, the easier hosting events will be for you!

4 Festive Menus for Special Occasions

There are so many different events and gatherings that call for amazing appetizers. What better way to set the tone of any party than with a few showstoppers? Wow all your friends, family, and coworkers with your keto creations, regardless of the occasion.

Game Day

- Sriracha Wings (page 20)

- Pimento Cheese (page 113)

- Pigs in a Blanket (page 18)

- Cheesy Chicken Taquitos (page 34)

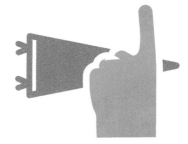

TIP: For the Pimento Cheese, plate the cheese in the center with keto-friendly crackers and regular crackers forming each side of a football or basketball around it.

Dinner Party

- Maple Bacon-Wrapped Brussels Sprouts (page 30)

- Salmon Salad Sushi Bites (page 49)

- Crab and Artichoke Dip (page 100)

- Cheddar-Chive Biscuits (page 69)

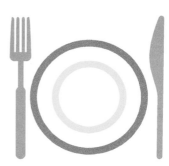

TIP: Stick individual toothpicks through the top of each Maple Bacon-Wrapped Brussels Sprout so your dinner guests can easily grab them.

Movie Night In

- Savory Party Mix (page 45)

- Peanut Butter Cookies (page 41)

- Sesame Seed Crackers (page 90)

- Creamy Spinach Dip (page 107)

TIP: Serve the Creamy Spinach Dip in a vessel where you can keep it at a warm temperature; that way it retains its silky-smooth texture and allows any type of chip or cracker to scoop it easily.

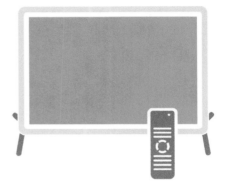

Holiday Luncheon

- Chocolate-Almond Fat Bombs (page 59)

- Toasty Granola Bars (page 54)

- Antipasto Skewers (page 16)

- Sun-Dried Tomato Cream Cheese (page 97)

TIP: The holidays are such a festive period. Try adorning your Chocolate-Almond Fat Bombs with unsweetened shredded coconut to give them a nice snowy touch!

Essential Kitchen Equipment

Before we jump into the recipes, there are a few essential kitchen items that will make your work much easier.

Sheet Pan: These are great for cooking in volume and also good for providing the crispy, roasted goodness (e.g., Sriracha Wings, page 20) that party-goers crave.

Mixing Bowl: This is absolutely essential because this is where all the magic happens! Mix together your favorite creamy dips and cheesy spreads in a good-size mixing bowl before transporting them to their final decorative destination.

Toothpicks: When serving individual finger foods such as fat bombs or Cheesy Baked Meatballs (page 26), the easiest way to ensure your guests can grab what they want without touching every item is to use toothpicks. Your toothpicks can be as plain or as festive as you want.

Skillet: This is necessary for any shallow frying you may want to do. My skillet of choice is a cast-iron skillet; it retains heat and gives an even cook to all items. Coat the bottom of the skillet with your favorite healthy fat, like avocado oil, and use it to fry your Zucchini Fritters (page 29) or "Latkes" with Sour Cream (page 38) to perfection.

Parchment Paper: I've been using parchment paper a lot more than aluminum foil lately. It's just so versatile. You can line your sheet pan with it in preparation for your fat bombs, or even line a loaf pan for easy removal of your Almond-Flour Bread (page 76) or Sour Cream "Corn" Bread (page 73).

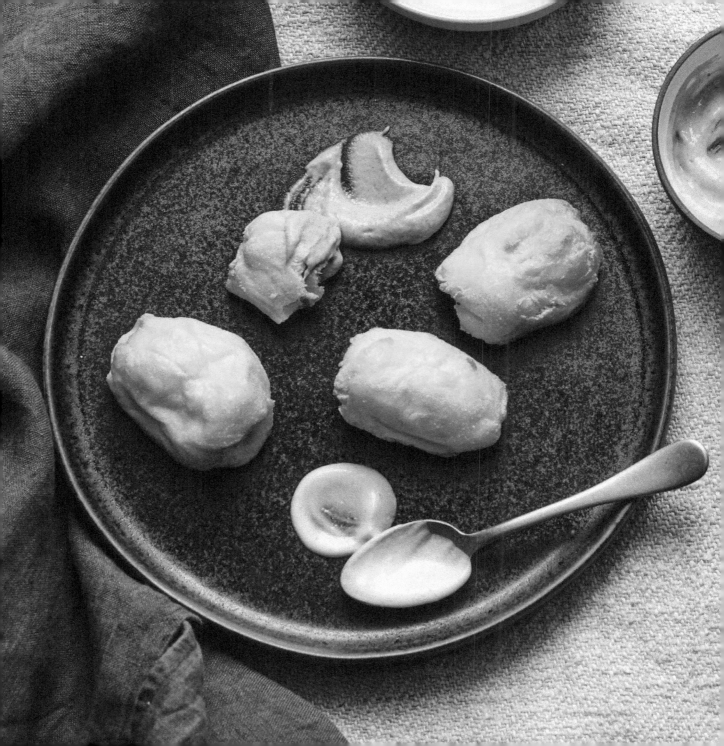

CHAPTER 2
Potluck Favorites

Antipasto Skewers

NUT-FREE

SERVES: 12 | **PREP TIME:** 10 minutes

These skewers are just as fun to make as they are to eat! The marinated mozzarella balls, grape tomatoes, various olives, and deli meats are sure to impress your guests. These savory sticks will be the perfect vibrant touch to any party or gathering. I prefer to use thick-cut deli meats, since they stay on the skewer better than a thinly sliced version.

12 Kalamata olives

12 thick-cut salami slices

12 pimento-stuffed green olives

12 marinated baby mozzarella balls

12 thick-cut summer sausage slices

12 grape tomatoes

1. On a 7-inch wooden or bamboo knotted skewer, thread the ingredients in this order: Kalamata olive, salami (end to end), green olive, mozzarella ball, summer sausage (end to end), and tomato.

2. Repeat with the remaining skewers. Plate and serve the skewers, or store in an airtight container in the refrigerator until ready to serve.

■ **VARIATION TIP:** Drizzle the finished product with balsamic vinegar for an extra flavor boost.

PER SERVING (1 SKEWER): Calories: 204; Fat: 16g; Protein: 12g; Total carbs: 2g; Fiber: 0g; Net carbs: 2g

MACROS: Fat: 72%; Protein: 24%; Carbs: 4%

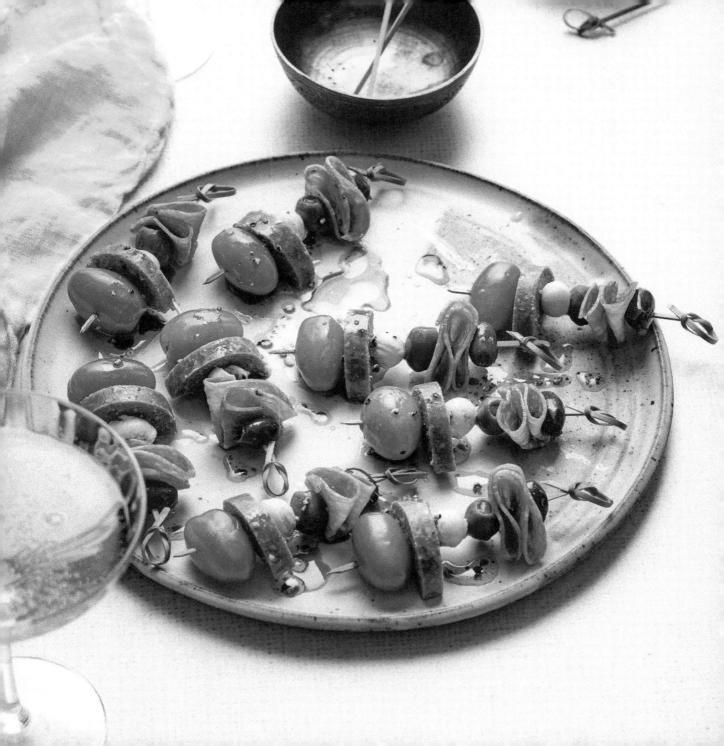

Pigs in a Blanket

SERVES: 9 | **PREP TIME:** 10 minutes, plus 15 minutes to rest | **COOK TIME:** 25 minutes

Who doesn't love pigs in a blanket? You can usually find these little sausages wrapped in biscuits, croissants, pancakes, or any other pastry dough. The "blanket" in this recipe is modified to be keto compliant using mozzarella cheese and coconut flour. These delicious bites will have your guests coming back to the table!

2 cups grated mozzarella cheese

2½ ounces (5 tablespoons) cream cheese

½ cup coconut flour

1 large egg

½ teaspoon garlic salt

6 smoked sausages, cut into thirds (check the carb count)

1. Preheat the oven to 350°F. Line a sheet pan with parchment paper.

2. In a large, microwave-safe bowl, combine the mozzarella cheese and cream cheese. Microwave on high power in 20-second increments until the mozzarella is melted and smooth. Remove from the microwave. Mix together.

3. Add the flour, egg, and garlic salt. Using your hands, mix well, then form into a ball of dough. Let rest for about 15 minutes.

4. Divide the dough in half repeatedly until you have 18 sections. Using damp hands, roll a dough section into a ball. Place the ball in the palm of your hand, and flatten it out.

5. Place a sausage on the dough, and wrap the dough around the sausage completely. Place on the prepared sheet pan and repeat with the remaining sausage and dough.

6. Transfer the sheet pan to the oven, and bake, rotating the pan halfway through, for 20 to 25 minutes, or until the pigs in a blanket are golden brown. Remove from the oven. Serve warm.

PER SERVING (2 PIGS IN A BLANKET): Calories: 212; Fat: 16g; Protein: 11g; Total carbs: 5g; Fiber: 2g; Net carbs: 3g

MACROS: Fat: 70%; Protein: 20%; Carbs: 10%

Sriracha Wings

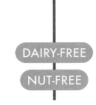

SERVES: 5 | **PREP TIME:** 10 minutes | **COOK TIME:** 1 hour

These Sriracha chicken wings are sure to bring the heat! Wings are the perfect keto appetizer because they contain a great amount of both fat and protein. What's even better is that the skin on chicken wings gets nice and crispy without any added flour—so you can skip the carbs but not the flavor. Bold, fiery Sriracha on top of these crispy wings will definitely score you all the points.

1 (2½-pound) package chicken wings (20 to 22 wings), patted dry
1 tablespoon garlic powder
1 tablespoon baking powder
½ teaspoon kosher salt
¼ teaspoon freshly ground black pepper

½ cup Sriracha
1 teaspoon sesame oil
1 teaspoon soy sauce
1 teaspoon brown erythritol blend
2 tablespoons sesame seeds

1. Preheat the oven to 425°F. Line a sheet pan with parchment paper.

2. Spread the chicken wings out on the prepared sheet pan.

3. In a small bowl, combine the garlic powder, baking powder, salt, and pepper.

4. Sprinkle half of the mixture evenly on top of the chicken wings. Flip, and sprinkle with the other half of the mixture.

5. Transfer the sheet pan to the oven, and bake, flipping the wings halfway through, for 50 minutes. Remove from the oven, leaving the oven on.

6. In a medium bowl, whisk together the Sriracha, oil, soy sauce, and erythritol blend.

7. Dip the wings in the mixture to coat evenly and place them back on the sheet pan.

8. Return the sheet pan to the oven, and bake for 10 minutes. Remove from the oven.

9. Garnish with the sesame seeds, and serve.

■ **VARIATION TIP:** Add a tablespoon of sweetener of your choice to transform these into sweet and spicy wings.

PER SERVING (4 WINGS): Calories: 471; Fat: 33g; Protein: 41g; Total carbs: 3g; Fiber: 1g; Net carbs: 2g

MACROS: Fat: 63%; Protein: 35%; Carbs: 2%

Bacon-Blue Cheese Deviled Eggs

NUT-FREE

SERVES: 12 | **PREP TIME:** 15 minutes

Deviled eggs are a standard potluck favorite. Eggs, cheese, and bacon are all staples in the keto diet because they contain a great amount of both fat and protein. These deviled eggs combine all three and take it up a notch with a pungent kick of blue cheese.

6 hard-boiled large eggs, peeled
¼ cup mayonnaise
½ teaspoon Dijon mustard

¼ cup blue cheese crumbles
Freshly ground black pepper
6 bacon slices, cooked and chopped

1. Halve each of the eggs lengthwise. Carefully remove the yolks, and put them in a medium bowl. Place the whites, hollow-side up, on a plate.

2. Using a fork, mash the yolks.

3. Add the mayonnaise, mustard, and most of the blue cheese, reserving about a tablespoon. Stir until well mixed. Season with pepper.

4. Spoon the yolk mixture back into the egg white hollows.

5. Top each egg half with the bacon and remaining blue cheese crumbles. Store in an airtight container in the refrigerator for up to 1 day.

■ **PREP TIP:** Save time by boiling your eggs ahead. Store them in the refrigerator until it's time to prepare this dish.

PER SERVING (1 DEVILED EGG): Calories: 104; Fat: 9g; Protein: 6g; Total carbs: 1g; Fiber: 0g; Net carbs: 1g

MACROS: Fat: 74%; Protein: 23%; Carbs: 3%

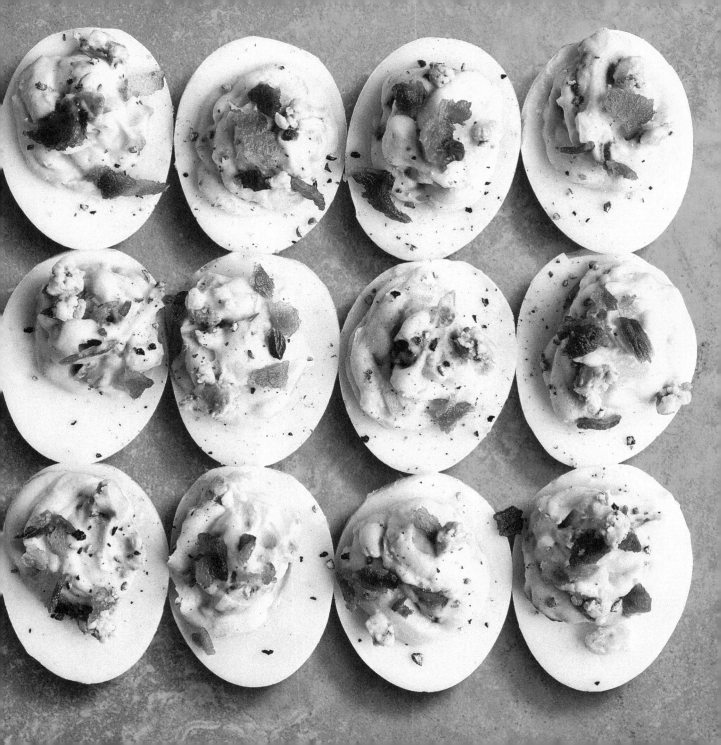

Sausage- and Spinach-Stuffed Mushrooms

SERVES: 15 | **PREP TIME:** 15 minutes | **COOK TIME:** 35 to 40 minutes

Stuffed mushrooms are an extremely versatile appetizer since they can be filled with a variety of keto-friendly ingredients. If the filling is quite heavy, you can pair a few of these with a side salad to serve as a meal. The mushrooms are stuffed with spicy sausage, a blend of cheeses, and fresh spinach. They're a nice balance of creamy and savory and are sure to wake up your taste buds.

15 whole button mushrooms, or cremini mushrooms, cleaned (stems reserved)

3 tablespoons unsalted butter

2 tablespoons finely chopped onion

2 garlic cloves, minced

¼ teaspoon kosher salt

1 cup fresh spinach, chopped

8 ounces spicy pork sausage

1 tablespoon gluten-free Worcestershire sauce

1 tablespoon chopped fresh parsley

⅓ cup shredded Parmesan cheese, plus more for garnish

½ cup shredded Fontina cheese

1. Preheat the oven to 400°F. Line a sheet pan with parchment paper.

2. Finely chop the reserved mushroom stems.

3. In a sauté pan or skillet, melt the butter over medium to medium-high heat. Add the onion, garlic, mushroom stems, and salt. Cook for 7 to 10 minutes, or until the onion is translucent and soft and the liquid from the mushroom stems is almost gone.

4. Stir in the spinach and cook for about 2 minutes, or just until the spinach wilts. Remove from the heat. Let cool.

5. To make the filling, in a medium bowl, combine the sausage, Worcestershire sauce, parsley, and cooled spinach mixture. Add the Parmesan and Fontina cheeses. Mix until thoroughly combined.

6. Stuff each mushroom cap with about 1 tablespoon of filling, depending on its size. The filling should be heaping.

7. Arrange the stuffed mushrooms on the prepared sheet pan. Sprinkle the mushrooms with a little Parmesan cheese.

8. Transfer the sheet pan to the oven, and bake for 20 to 25 minutes, or until the mushrooms have cooked through and browned. Remove from the oven. Serve warm or at room temperature.

PER SERVING (1 STUFFED MUSHROOM): Calories: 103; Fat: 9g; Protein: 4g; Total carbs: 2g; Fiber: 0g; Net carbs: 2g

MACROS: Fat: 76%; Protein: 17%; Carbs: 7%

Cheesy Baked Meatballs

SERVES: 12 | **PREP TIME:** 20 minutes | **COOK TIME:** 40 to 45 minutes

The tang from the tomatoes and chiles pairs perfectly with the salty Parmesan and creamy mozzarella. Without a doubt, you've got an absolutely irresistible appetizer. Serve with toothpicks or mini skewers for easy picking.

¼ cup olive oil, plus more for greasing the baking dish

2 garlic cloves, minced

1 (10-ounce) can diced tomatoes with green chiles

1 (8-ounce) can tomato sauce

1 teaspoon kosher salt, divided

¼ teaspoon freshly ground black pepper, divided

1½ pounds ground beef

½ cup crushed pork skins

¾ cup grated Parmesan cheese, divided

1 large egg

½ teaspoon garlic powder

½ cup grated mozzarella cheese

1. Preheat the oven to 375°F. Lightly grease a 9-by-13-inch baking dish.

2. In a medium pot, heat the oil over medium-low heat. Add the garlic, and sauté for 1 to 2 minutes. Reduce the heat to low. Add the diced tomatoes with their juices, tomato sauce, ½ teaspoon of salt, and ⅛ teaspoon of pepper. Cook, stirring occasionally, while you make the meatballs.

3. In a large bowl, combine the ground beef, pork skins, ½ cup of Parmesan cheese, the egg, garlic powder, and the remaining salt and pepper. Mix well, scoop, and roll into 24 balls about 1½ inches in diameter. Place the meatballs side by side in the prepared baking dish.

Continued ›››

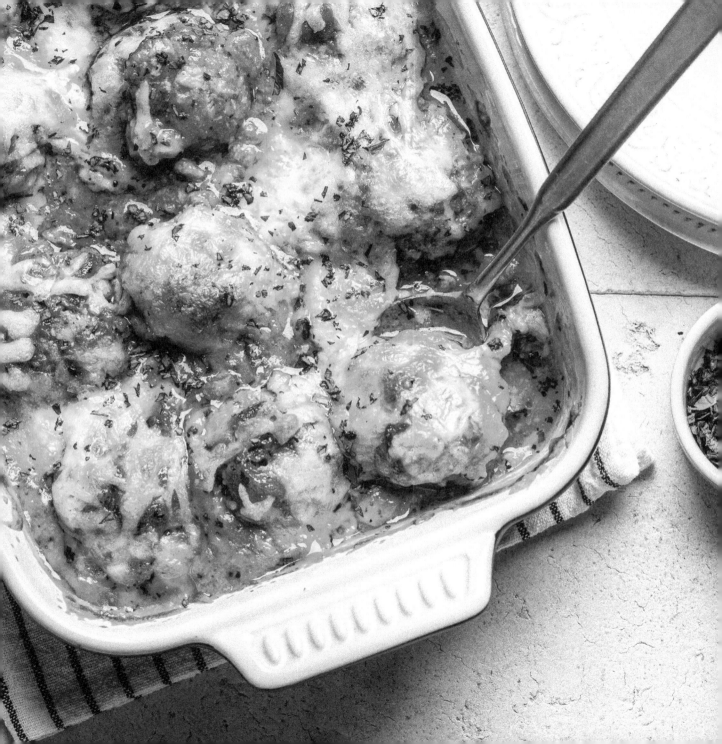

4. Transfer the baking dish to the oven, and bake for 20 minutes. Remove from the oven, cover the meatballs with the sauce, and top with the mozzarella cheese.

5. Return the baking dish to the oven, and bake for 20 minutes; cover lightly with aluminum foil if the cheese begins to get too brown. Remove from the oven.

6. Garnish with the remaining ¼ cup of Parmesan cheese. Serve.

■ **PREP TIP:** This recipe freezes well, so feel free to make extras and heat them up at a later date.

PER SERVING (2 MEATBALLS): Calories: 265; Fat: 21g; Protein: 16g; Total carbs: 3g; Fiber: 0g; Net carbs: 3g

MACROS: Fat: 70%; Protein: 26%; Carbs: 4%

Zucchini Fritters

SERVES: 8 | **PREP TIME:** 20 minutes | **COOK TIME:** 15 minutes

Growing up, corn fritters were one of my favorite appetizers from a local restaurant. Obviously it would be hard to stay within carb limits with corn, so zucchini is a great alternative. As long as you make sure the zucchini is thoroughly dried, you will have scrumptious, savory fritters for your guests to devour.

2 cups grated zucchini
½ teaspoon kosher salt
2 large eggs, beaten
½ teaspoon baking powder
½ cup almond flour

2 tablespoons coconut flour
¼ cup grated Parmesan cheese
½ cup peanut oil
½ cup sour cream
2 tablespoons chopped fresh chives

1. Line a plate with paper towels. Put the zucchini in a medium bowl, and sprinkle with the salt. Set aside for 5 minutes. Transfer to a colander. Squeeze dry with more paper towels. Once the zucchini is as dry as possible, return to the bowl.

2. Add the eggs, baking powder, almond flour, coconut flour, and cheese. Mix until well combined and a batter forms.

3. In a small skillet, heat the oil over high heat. Pour ¼ cup of batter per fritter into the hot skillet, and spread into flat pancakes. Cook for 3 minutes. Flip, and cook for another 3 minutes. Transfer to the prepared plate to drain. Repeat until all the batter has been used. You should have about 8 fritters.

4. Top each fritter with 1 tablespoon of sour cream, and sprinkle with the chives.

■ **PREP TIP:** Try a cheesecloth to squeeze the zucchini dry. The drier, the better.

PER SERVING (1 FRITTER): Calories: 218; Fat: 21g; Protein: 4g; Total carbs: 3g; Fiber: 1g; Net carbs: 2g

MACROS: Fat: 86%; Protein: 8%; Carbs: 6%

Maple Bacon-Wrapped Brussels Sprouts

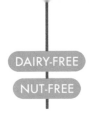

SERVES: 20 | **PREP TIME:** 10 minutes | **COOK TIME:** 30 minutes

Interestingly enough, I did not have my first taste of Brussels sprouts until after college. They'd always been portrayed in cartoons as the vegetable no child wanted to eat. Boy, was I missing out! When cooked properly, Brussels sprouts have a sweet and nutty flavor that is absolutely delightful. In this recipe, that flavor is enhanced by the addition of savory bacon. This sweet and salty pairing is sure to be a hit at any party.

20 Brussels sprouts
¾ cup sugar-free maple-flavored
   syrup, divided
20 bacon slices, cut in half
2 cups mayonnaise

2 teaspoons Sriracha
2 teaspoons Dijon mustard
1 teaspoon kosher salt
1 teaspoon freshly ground black pepper

1. Preheat the oven to 400°F. Line a sheet pan with parchment paper.

2. Trim the ends off the Brussels sprouts, remove any wilted leaves, and halve the sprouts lengthwise.

3. Drizzle ¼ cup of syrup on the bacon slices.

4. Roll each Brussels sprout half with a piece of bacon, syrup-side out. Secure with a toothpick.

5. Place the sprouts on the prepared sheet pan, leaving a little room between each sprout.

6. Transfer the sheet pan to the oven, and bake, rotating the pan halfway through, for 30 minutes, or until the bacon is crispy and the Brussels sprouts are fork tender. Remove from the oven.

7. In a small bowl, combine the mayonnaise, remaining ½ cup of syrup, the Sriracha, mustard, salt, and pepper. Serve with the Brussels sprouts.

■ **INGREDIENT TIP:** Try using thick-cut bacon to increase the bacon flavor on each sprout.

PER SERVING (2 MAPLE BACON-WRAPPED BRUSSEL SPROUTS): Calories: 240; Fat: 21g; Protein: 5g; Total carbs: 4g; Fiber: 1g; Net carbs: 1g;

MACROS: Fat: 87%; Protein: 9%; Carbs: 4%

Pizza Pull-Apart Bread

SERVES: 8 | **PREP TIME:** 15 minutes, plus 30 minutes to chill | **COOK TIME:** 30 minutes

Pull-apart bread is most definitely a crowd-pleaser. Combining the classic flavors of pizza, this dish is an instant hit. The options are endless since you can choose to add more than just pepperoni. Jazz it up with your favorite pizza toppings and serve with a variety of dips!

Butter or nonstick cooking spray, for greasing

2½ cups grated mozzarella cheese

2 ounces (4 tablespoons) cream cheese

1¼ cups almond flour

2 tablespoons flaxseed meal

2 tablespoons coconut flour

2 large eggs

2 tablespoons whey protein isolate, unflavored

2 tablespoons finely grated Parmesan cheese

1 tablespoon baking powder

¼ teaspoon garlic salt

1 pound pork breakfast sausage, cooked and drained

30 pepperoni slices

1. Preheat the oven to 350°F. Grease a Bundt pan with butter or nonstick cooking spray.

2. In a microwave-safe dish, combine the mozzarella cheese and cream cheese. Microwave on high power in 20-second increments until the mozzarella is melted and smooth. Remove from the microwave. Mix together.

3. Add the almond flour, flaxseed meal, coconut flour, and eggs. Using your hands, mix together and then form the dough into a ball. Refrigerate for at least 30 minutes or more.

4. In a small bowl, combine the whey protein, Parmesan cheese, baking powder, and garlic salt.

5. Spread a piece of parchment paper on the countertop. Remove the dough from the refrigerator, and place it on the parchment. Divide the dough in half repeatedly until you have 32 equal portions, then roll each into a ball.

6. Roll each ball in the baking powder mixture.

7. Evenly place a quarter of the sausage and pepperoni in the bottom of the prepared Bundt pan, add 8 of the balls, and sprinkle in half of the Parmesan cheese mixture. Repeat, evenly adding the remaining sausage, pepperoni, balls, and cheese.

8. Transfer the Bundt pan to the oven, and bake for 30 minutes. Remove from the oven. Run a knife around the inside of the pan to make sure the bread will pull apart from the sides, then place a plate on top and flip over. If you think the bottom looks prettier, put another plate on the bread and flip over again so the bottom side is up.

PER SERVING (⅛ OF THE BREAD): Calories: 493; Fat: 39g; Protein: 29g; Total carbs: 8g; Fiber: 3g; Net carbs: 5g

MACROS: Fat: 70%; Protein: 24%; Carbs: 6%

Cheesy Chicken Taquitos

NUT-FREE

SERVES: 12 | **PREP TIME:** 15 minutes | **COOK TIME:** 15 minutes

Taquitos, also known as rolled tacos, are very popular here in Texas. In this recipe, the classic taco shell is replaced with slices of cheddar cheese. Cheese is surprisingly flexible once baked. Cook a batch of the delicious chicken filling, spoon onto the melted cheese slices, and get to rolling. These taquitos are full of flavor served with or without additional toppings.

12 large (deli-sliced) cheddar cheese slices

3 ounces (6 tablespoons) cream cheese

¼ cup tomato salsa

1 tablespoon freshly squeezed lime juice

1 teaspoon chili powder

1 teaspoon garlic salt

½ teaspoon freshly ground black pepper

2 cups shredded cooked chicken

¾ cup sour cream

1 or 2 scallions, both white and green parts, chopped

1. Preheat the oven to 375°F. Line 2 sheet pans with parchment paper.

2. Lay 6 cheddar cheese slices on each sheet pan an equal distance apart.

3. In a medium skillet, mix together the cream cheese, salsa, lime juice, chili powder, garlic salt, and pepper over medium heat.

4. Add the chicken, and mix until heated through. Remove from the heat.

5. Transfer the sheet pans to the oven, and bake for 6 to 10 minutes, or until the edges of the cheese are brown and bubbly. Remove from the oven. Let cool for a couple of minutes.

6. When the cheese is cool enough to handle, peel it off the parchment paper, and place it on a clean piece of parchment paper.

7. Divide the chicken mixture onto each piece of cheese, and wrap tightly. Transfer the taquitos to a serving dish.

8. Top each with 1 tablespoon of sour cream, and sprinkle with the scallions.

■ VARIATION TIP: You can use various types of sliced cheeses for different flavor profiles.

PER SERVING (1 TAQUITO): Calories: 206; Fat: 16g; Protein: 14g; Total carbs: 2g; Fiber: 0g; Net carbs: 2g

MACROS: Fat: 68%; Protein: 28%; Carbs: 4%

Herbed Mozzarella Sticks

SERVES: 8 | **PREP TIME:** 10 minutes | **COOK TIME:** 20 minutes

Mozzarella sticks are ooey, gooey, and downright delicious. This recipe swaps out the standard carb-heavy breadcrumbs for finely grated Parmesan cheese—which, when fried, creates a light, crispy coating ideal for mozzarella sticks. Serve these warm with low-carb marinara or any dipping sauce of your choice.

½ cup peanut oil

1 cup very finely grated Parmesan cheese

1 tablespoon Italian seasoning

½ teaspoon garlic salt

8 sticks full-fat string cheese, halved horizontally

2 large eggs, beaten

1. In a small skillet, heat the oil over high heat. Line a plate with paper towels.

2. Meanwhile, in a small bowl, combine the Parmesan cheese, Italian seasoning, and garlic salt.

3. Dredge each mozzarella stick first in the beaten eggs and then in the cheese-and-herb mixture, rolling the sticks so they are fully coated.

4. Carefully slip 3 or 4 sticks into the hot oil. Cook for about 3 minutes, or until all sides are golden brown. Transfer to the prepared plate to drain for a few minutes. Repeat with the remaining cheese sticks. Remove from the heat. Serve warm.

■ **INGREDIENT TIP:** If you don't have peanut oil, avocado oil is also excellent for frying.

PER SERVING (1 MOZZARELLA STICK): Calories: 200; Fat: 16g; Protein: 11g; Total carbs: 3g; Fiber: 0g; Net carbs: 3g

MACROS: Fat: 71%; Protein: 24%; Carbs: 5%

Caprese-Stuffed Avocados

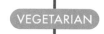

SERVES: 8 | **PREP TIME:** 10 minutes

Caprese is a popular Italian flavor combination that is usually seen on pizzas and in salads. The main ingredients are tomatoes, mozzarella, and basil; sometimes a balsamic glaze or reduction is added. The word "reduction" sometimes refers to an ingredient in a caramelized state, which would categorize it as non-keto. Here, we use balsamic vinegar because it is much lower in carbs and sugar.

1 cup small mozzarella balls, or
   bocconcini, halved
⅔ cup halved cherry tomatoes
¼ cup pesto
2 teaspoons garlic salt

4 ripe avocados, halved and pitted
3 tablespoons balsamic vinegar
   (optional)
Freshly ground black pepper
¼ cup chopped fresh basil leaves

1. In a medium bowl, combine the mozzarella balls, tomatoes, pesto, and garlic salt.

2. Divide the mixture between the avocado halves.

3. Drizzle with the vinegar, if using. Season with pepper.

4. Garnish with the basil.

PER SERVING (1 STUFFED AVOCADO HALF): Calories: 249; Fat: 22g; Protein: 6g; Total carbs: 10g; Fiber: 7g; Net carbs: 3g

MACROS: Fat: 75%; Protein: 10%; Carbs: 15%

"Latkes" with Sour Cream

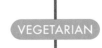

SERVES: 12 | **PREP TIME:** 15 minutes | **COOK TIME:** 45 minutes

A standard latke is basically a potato pancake. In this recipe, potatoes are replaced with coarsely chopped cauliflower, which has proven to be a pretty adequate keto-friendly substitute for potatoes in many recipes. Once combined with other ingredients to make these "latkes," they are fried in olive oil and topped with a creamy, cool dollop of sour cream.

1 (2-pound) head cauliflower, stems trimmed and florets coarsely chopped

4 tablespoons olive oil, divided

½ teaspoon freshly ground black pepper

½ teaspoon garlic powder

½ teaspoon kosher salt

½ cup grated mozzarella cheese

½ cup grated cheddar cheese

2 large eggs

3 tablespoons coconut flour

2 tablespoons mayonnaise

1 cup sour cream

2 scallions, both white and green parts, chopped

1. Preheat the oven to 450°F. Line a sheet pan with parchment paper.

2. Put the cauliflower in a gallon-size resealable bag. Add 2 tablespoons of oil, seal, and massage and turn the bag to coat the cauliflower.

3. Spread the cauliflower out in a single layer on the prepared sheet pan. Season with the pepper, garlic powder, and salt.

4. Transfer the sheet pan to the oven, and roast for 30 minutes. Remove from the oven. Let the cauliflower cool.

5. When the cauliflower is cool enough to handle, coarsely chop it. Transfer it to a medium bowl.

6. Add the mozzarella cheese, cheddar cheese, eggs, flour, and mayonnaise. Mix well.

7. In a medium nonstick skillet, heat the remaining 2 tablespoons of oil over medium heat. Line a plate with paper towels.

8. Working in batches and being careful not to crowd the skillet, use a large spoon to scoop the cauliflower mixture into the skillet and pat down into patties. Cook for 2 to 3 minutes, or until golden brown on one side.

9. Flip the patties, and cook 2 minutes on the other side. Remove from the heat. Transfer to the prepared plate.

10. Top each latke with a spoonful of sour cream, and garnish with the scallions.

■ VARIATION TIP: Top the "latkes" with cheddar cheese and bacon for another savory twist.

PER SERVING (1 OR 2 LATKES, DEPENDING ON SIZE): Calories: 158; Fat: 14g; Protein: 5g; Total carbs: 5g; Fiber: 2g; Net carbs: 3g

MACROS: Fat: 77%; Protein: 12%; Carbs: 11%

Orange Cream Ice Pops

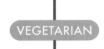 VEGETARIAN

MAKES: 8 pops | **PREP TIME:** 5 minutes, plus 3 hours to freeze

Do you remember the creamy orange pops from your childhood? The classic blend of orange and vanilla was honestly divine. These orange cream pops are a pretty spot-on replica, minus the vibrant orange food coloring, of course. Since these need to be kept frozen, bring them out towards the end of your event, and let your guests wind down with a cool, refreshing treat.

2 cups unsweetened almond milk
¾ cup cream cheese, softened
3 tablespoons egg white protein powder
2 teaspoons orange extract

2 teaspoons pure vanilla extract
½ teaspoon stevia
Pinch sea salt

1. Put the almond milk, cream cheese, protein powder, orange extract, vanilla extract, stevia, and salt in a blender. Blend until the mixture is very smooth.

2. Pour into 8 ice pop molds, freeze for at least 3 hours, and serve.

■ **INGREDIENT TIP:** Make sure your cream cheese is at room temperature to ensure the best blend. This will help you avoid any lumps in the final ice cream pops.

PER SERVING (1 POP): Calories: 97; Fat: 8g; Protein: 4g; Total carbs: 2g; Fiber: 0g; Net carbs: 2g

MACROS: Fat: 74%; Protein: 19%; Carbs: 7%

Peanut Butter Cookies

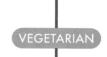

VEGETARIAN

MAKES: 20 cookies | **PREP TIME:** 10 minutes | **COOK TIME:** 15 minutes

Want something sweet to place on the table? Look no further! These peanut butter cookies are sweetened with xylitol and use a mixture of almond flour and protein powder as the base. All the ingredients are keto friendly and create the perfect soft and chewy cookie.

½ cup natural peanut butter
5 tablespoons unsalted butter
1 tablespoon heavy cream
1 large egg
1½ cups almond flour

½ cup xylitol
¼ cup egg white protein powder
1 teaspoon baking powder
¼ teaspoon baking soda

1. Preheat the oven to 350°F. Line a sheet pan with parchment paper.

2. In a large bowl, beat together the peanut butter, butter, cream, and egg until creamy and smooth.

3. Stir in the flour, xylitol, protein powder, baking powder, and baking soda. Form the mixture into about 20 balls of dough.

4. Place the dough balls on the prepared sheet pan. Using a fork, press down the balls to create a crosshatch design.

5. Transfer the sheet pan to the oven, and bake for about 15 minutes, or until the cookies are crisp and lightly brown. Remove from the oven. Let cool on a wire rack. Refrigerate in a sealed container for up to 1 week.

■ **VARIATION TIP:** Add sugar-free chocolate chips to offer your guests variety.

PER SERVING (1 COOKIE): Calories: 136; Fat: 10g; Protein: 4g; Total carbs: 8g; Fiber: 2g; Net carbs: 1g;

MACROS: Fat: 76%; Protein: 14%; Carbs: 10%

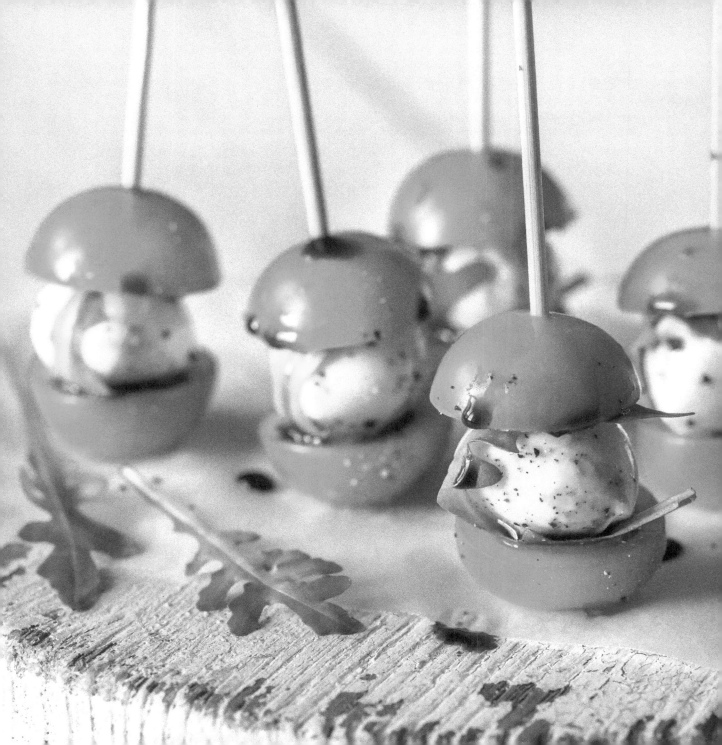

CHAPTER 3
Pass-Arounds

Spicy Barbecue Pecans

SERVES: 8 | **PREP TIME:** 15 minutes | **COOK TIME:** 20 minutes

Pecans are one of the best nuts to eat on the keto diet. They contain a substantial amount of fat and very minimal carbs. The pecans are toasted, salted, and seasoned to perfection. They make for a great salty, crunchy snack, and you can prepack them into individual party bags or cups for easy grabbing.

2½ tablespoons unsalted butter, melted

1 tablespoon gluten-free Worcestershire Sauce

1 tablespoon tamari, or gluten-free soy sauce

1 teaspoon kosher salt

½ teaspoon chili powder

½ teaspoon garlic powder

¼ teaspoon cayenne

¼ teaspoon dry mustard

2 cups pecan halves

1. Preheat the oven to 325°F. Line a sheet pan with parchment paper.

2. In a medium bowl, combine the butter, Worcestershire sauce, tamari, salt, chili powder, garlic powder, cayenne, and mustard.

3. Add the pecans, and toss to coat well. Pour the coated pecans onto the prepared sheet pan, and spread into a single layer.

4. Transfer the sheet pan to the oven, and bake, stirring once halfway through, for 18 to 20 minutes. Keep a close eye on the pecans to ensure they don't burn. Remove from the oven. Spread the pecan halves on paper towels to cool completely before packing in an airtight container for storage.

■ **VARIATION TIP:** This recipe also works well with peanuts, walnuts, and almonds.

PER SERVING (¼ CUP PECANS): Calories: 207; Fat: 21g; Protein: 3g; Total carbs: 4g; Fiber: 3g; Net carbs: 1g

MACROS: Fat: 87%; Protein: 5%; Carbs: 8%

Savory Party Mix

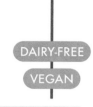

SERVES: 12 | **PREP TIME:** 5 minutes | **COOK TIME:** 20 minutes

Skip the rice- or corn-based cereal. This party mix is loaded with nuts and seeds that are packed with healthy fats. The seasoning combo gives them an amazing flavor profile that will have your guests munching endlessly.

½ cup pecans

½ cup cashews

½ cup pistachios

½ cup peanuts

½ cup almonds

½ cup pumpkin seeds

½ cup sunflower seeds

2 teaspoons onion powder

1 teaspoon garlic powder

½ teaspoon kosher salt

2 tablespoons olive oil

1. Preheat the oven to 350°F. Line a sheet pan with parchment paper.

2. In a large mixing bowl, combine the pecans, cashews, pistachios, peanuts, almonds, pumpkin seeds, and sunflower seeds. Stir in the onion powder, garlic powder, and salt.

3. Pour in the oil. Toss well to thoroughly coat the nuts and seeds with the oil. Spread the mixture out in a single layer on the prepared sheet pan.

4. Transfer the sheet pan to the oven, and bake for 10 minutes. Remove from the oven, leaving the oven on. Stir well, and return the mix to the oven to bake for 10 more minutes. Remove from the oven. Let cool completely before serving.

■ **VARIATION TIP:** This recipe can easily be converted into a sweet mix by swapping out the onion powder and garlic powder for erythritol and cinnamon.

PER SERVING: Calories: 245; Fat: 22g; Protein: 8g; Total carbs: 9g; Fiber: 3g; Net carbs: 6g

MACROS: Fat: 74%; Protein: 12%; Carbs: 14%

Oven-Fried Green Tomatoes with Avocado Ranch

SERVES: 6 | **PREP TIME:** 15 minutes, plus 1 hour to chill | **COOK TIME:** 10 minutes

Fried green tomatoes are a Southern classic. Green tomatoes are simply unripened tomatoes—they have a slightly tangy flavor in comparison to the natural subtle sweetness of a red tomato. This recipe uses grated Parmesan and almond flour for the breading. Pop them in the oven, and get ready for golden, crispy goodness! Don't forget the creamy avocado ranch for dipping.

FOR THE AVOCADO RANCH

½ cup mayonnaise
½ cup unsweetened almond milk
⅓ cup mashed avocado
1 garlic clove, peeled
2 teaspoons gluten-free
    Worcestershire sauce
1 teaspoon Creole mustard
½ teaspoon kosher salt
¼ teaspoon onion powder
1½ teaspoons dried parsley
½ teaspoon Italian seasoning

FOR THE FRIED GREEN TOMATOES

½ cup grated Parmesan cheese
¼ cup almond flour
¼ teaspoon freshly ground black pepper
¼ teaspoon garlic powder
¼ teaspoon paprika
¼ teaspoon kosher salt
⅛ teaspoon cayenne
1 tablespoon unsweetened almond milk
1 large egg, lightly beaten
3 green tomatoes, sliced

TO MAKE THE AVOCADO RANCH

1. Put the mayonnaise, almond milk, avocado, garlic, Worcestershire sauce, mustard, salt, and onion powder in a blender. Blend on high speed until smooth.

2. Add the parsley and Italian seasoning. Stir to combine, or blend on low speed until just mixed. Refrigerate for at least 1 hour before serving. Store in an airtight container or jar for up to 3 days.

TO MAKE THE FRIED GREEN TOMATOES

1. Preheat the oven to 425°F. Line a sheet pan with parchment paper.

2. In a small bowl, combine the cheese, flour, pepper, garlic powder, paprika, salt, and cayenne.

3. In a medium bowl, whisk together the almond milk and egg to combine.

4. One at a time, dip the tomato slices into the egg mixture, then dredge in the Parmesan-flour mixture, coating both sides well.

5. Place the coated tomato slices on the prepared sheet pan.

6. Transfer the sheet pan to the oven, and bake for about 5 minutes, or until the tomatoes are golden brown.

7. Flip the slices over, and bake for 5 more minutes. Remove from the oven.

8. Serve the tomatoes immediately with the avocado ranch.

■ **INGREDIENT TIP:** Use Parmesan cheese that comes in a canister; it's finely grated and yields the best result.

PER SERVING: Calories: 240; Fat: 21g; Protein: 6g; Total carbs: 8g; Fiber: 2g; Net carbs: 6g

MACROS: Fat: 77%; Protein: 10%; Carbs: 13%

Jalapeño Cheese Fudge

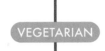

Don't let the name fool you! Despite this dish being called fudge, there isn't any chocolate in this recipe; think of it more as a cheesy soufflé. This recipe has a nice golden caramelized top and a flavorful spicy bottom. Once it's baked, cut into squares and serve on a festive platter. It can be enjoyed warm or at room temperature.

Nonstick cooking spray

6 ounces pickled sliced jalapeño peppers, drained and roughly chopped

1 pound mild or medium cheddar cheese, grated

1 pound Monterey Jack cheese, grated

3 extra-large eggs, beaten

¼ cup heavy cream

2 tablespoons unsweetened almond milk

¼ teaspoon garlic powder

⅛ teaspoon onion powder

1. Preheat the oven to 350°F. Lightly coat a 9-by-9-inch baking dish with cooking spray.

2. Spread the jalapeños in a single layer across the bottom of the prepared baking dish.

3. In a large bowl, combine the cheddar cheese, Monterey Jack cheese, eggs, cream, almond milk, garlic powder, and onion powder. (I find it easiest to use my hands.) Pour over the jalapeños, and spread evenly.

4. Transfer the baking dish to the oven, and bake for 30 to 35 minutes, or until the fudge is golden brown and bubbly. Remove from the oven. Let cool completely in the dish before cutting into 16 pieces. It's best served slightly warm or at room temperature.

PER SERVING (1 PIECE): Calories: 254; Fat: 21g; Protein: 15g; Total carbs: 2g; Fiber: 0g; Net carbs: 2g

MACROS: Fat: 72%; Protein: 25%; Carbs: 3%

Salmon Salad Sushi Bites

DAIRY-FREE
NUT-FREE

SERVES: 4 to 6 | **PREP TIME:** 20 minutes

These salmon salad sushi bites are sure to be a hit with sushi lovers at any event. The salmon filling is the perfect pairing with fresh cucumbers. You can use canned salmon to make setting this up a breeze, or smoked salmon for a slightly smoky flavor. This recipe is a fan fave amongst all ages!

2 large cucumbers, peeled

8 ounces canned salmon, preferably sockeye, bones and skin removed

¼ cup mayonnaise

1 tablespoon sesame oil

2 teaspoons miso

1 teaspoon Sriracha, or other hot sauce

1 nori sheet, crumbled

½ ripe avocado, pitted, peeled, and thinly sliced

1. Cut the cucumbers into 1-inch segments. Using a spoon, scrape the seeds out of the center of each segment and discard. Place the cucumbers, center-side up, on a plate.

2. In a medium bowl, combine the salmon, mayonnaise, oil, miso, Sriracha, and nori. Mix until creamy.

3. Spoon the salmon mixture into the center of each cucumber segment, and top with a slice of avocado. Serve chilled.

■ **PREP TIP:** The stuffing can be made and stored one day in advance.

PER SERVING: Calories: 263; Fat: 21g; Protein: 12g; Total carbs: 8g; Fiber: 3g; Net carbs: 5g

MACROS: Fat: 70%; Protein: 18%; Carbs: 12%

Jalapeño Firecrackers

 NUT-FREE

SERVES: 8 | **PREP TIME:** 20 minutes | **COOK TIME:** 20 minutes

This dish is anything but ordinary! Most jalapeño poppers call for the standard bacon and cream cheese. This recipe takes it up a notch by adding sugar-free apricot preserves. It introduces a sweet element that will catch your guests by surprise. They are also grilled, which heightens the flavor of this sweet and spicy treat.

6 ounces cream cheese
¼ cup sugar-free apricot preserves
⅛ teaspoon red pepper flakes

8 (3- to 4-inch) jalapeño peppers, stemmed, halved, and seeded
16 bacon slices, at room temperature

1. Preheat the grill on low heat. Using aluminum foil, make a flat-bottom boat large enough to hold 16 jalapeño halves, or use a grill mat.

2. In a small bowl, mash together the cream cheese, apricot preserves, and red pepper flakes until well incorporated.

3. Using a butter knife, fill each of the jalapeño halves with the cream cheese mixture.

4. Starting at the stem end of the jalapeño, lay a slice of bacon lengthwise across the cream cheese down toward the pointed end, then wrap the bacon around the jalapeño all the way back to the stem end so the entire jalapeño is covered lengthwise. This keeps the cream cheese from bubbling out. Repeat with the remaining jalapeños and bacon slices.

5. Place the jalapeños, cream cheese–side down, on the foil boat or mat.

6. Transfer the foil boat to the oven and cook for 10 minutes. Flip, and cook for another 10 minutes. Remove from the oven.

■ VARIATION TIP: The slight tanginesss of sugar-free orange marmalade will yield a similar result.

PER SERVING (2 JALAPEÑO FIRECRACKERS): Calories: 166; Fat: 14g; Protein: 7g; Total carbs: 2g; Fiber: 0g; Net carbs: 2g

MACROS: Fat: 77%; Protein: 18%; Carbs: 5%

Caprese Salad Bites

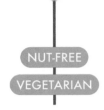

NUT-FREE

VEGETARIAN

SERVES: 6 | **PREP TIME:** 15 minutes

These vibrant mini skewers highlight key Italian flavors in one bite. The tomato and mozzarella complement each other effortlessly. The basil adds a fresh and herby element. Drizzling them with balsamic vinegar seals the deal with that slightly sweet yet tangy touch. Eye-catching and mouthwatering, these bites deserve to be front and center of any party!

12 cherry tomatoes, halved

12 bocconcini (small mozzarella balls), or 12 (1-ounce) mozzarella cubes

12 fresh basil leaves (or try arugula)

2 tablespoons olive oil

1 tablespoon balsamic vinegar

¼ teaspoon kosher salt

⅛ teaspoon freshly ground black pepper

1. Using a toothpick, spear 1 tomato half, then add 1 bocconcini.

2. Top the bocconcini with 1 basil leaf, then the second tomato half. Repeat the process with the remaining tomatoes, bocconcini, and basil.

3. Arrange the skewered bites on a tray.

4. Drizzle with the oil and vinegar. Season with the salt and pepper. Serve immediately, or chill for up to 24 hours.

■ **VARIATION TIP:** Use garlic salt in place of regular salt to add a savory flair to the dish.

PER SERVING (2 BITES): Calories: 109; Fat: 9g; Protein: 6g; Total carbs: 2g; Fiber: 0g; Net carbs: 2g

MACROS: Fat: 70%; Protein: 25%; Carbs: 5%

Smoked Salmon Wraps

MAKES: 12 wraps | **PREP TIME:** 20 minutes

Smoked salmon strips are the star of this recipe. Rolled in between each piece of smoked salmon is a delicious mixture of creamy cheese and fresh dill. These wraps are bursting with flavor and can be prepared ahead. Have thin strips of chives on hand to keep the wraps rolled and to provide a nice garnish.

¼ cup cottage cheese
¼ cup cream cheese
1 teaspoon freshly squeezed lemon juice
2 tablespoons finely chopped dill

Freshly ground black pepper
8 smoked Atlantic salmon strips
Chives, to tie around the wraps

1. In a small bowl, mix the cottage cheese, cream cheese, lemon juice, and dill for about 3 minutes, or until smooth and well blended. Season with pepper.

2. Lay the smoked salmon strips out on a clean work surface, and evenly divide the cheese mixture among them, placing the mixture at the far end of each strip.

3. Roll the first strip toward you and tie a chive around it to secure the wrap. Repeat with the remaining strips and cheese mixture. Refrigerate to chill before serving, and serve 2 wraps per person.

■ **PREP TIP:** These can be prepared ahead and stored for up to 2 days.

PER SERVING (2 WRAPS): Calories: 130; Fat: 6g; Protein: 16g; Total carbs: 0g; Fiber: 0g; Net carbs: 0g

MACROS: Fat: 47%; Protein: 50%; Carbs: 3%

Toasty Granola Bars

MAKES: 20 bars | **PREP TIME:** 10 minutes | **COOK TIME:** 15 minutes

These granola bars pack a powerful punch. Packed with protein, healthy fats, and various textures, your guests are sure to experience a flavor explosion with each bite. The shredded coconut and vanilla extract give a natural sweetness that is unmatched. They can be served alone or crumbled and placed alongside keto-friendly fruits and yogurt to make individual parfaits.

1 cup walnuts

1 cup unsweetened shredded coconut

1 cup slivered almonds

1 cup roasted sunflower seeds

¼ cup egg white protein powder

1 large egg

½ cup natural peanut butter

¼ cup coconut butter

1 tablespoon pure vanilla extract

1 teaspoon ground cinnamon

¼ teaspoon ground nutmeg

1. Preheat the oven to 350°F.

2. In a food processor, pulse the walnuts, coconut, almonds, sunflower seeds, and protein powder to coarsely chop the ingredients. Transfer to a large bowl.

3. Stir in the egg, peanut butter, coconut butter, vanilla, cinnamon, and nutmeg until well mixed.

4. Press the granola bar mixture into a 9-by-13-inch baking dish. Cut the mixture into 20 bars.

5. Transfer the baking dish to the oven, and bake for about 15 minutes, or until the bars are firm and golden. Remove from the oven. Let the bars cool in the baking dish. Refrigerate in a sealed container for up to 2 weeks.

PER SERVING (1 BAR): Calories: 197; Fat: 18g; Protein: 6g; Total carbs: 5g; Fiber: 3g; Net carbs: 2g

MACROS: Fat: 77%; Protein: 12%; Carbs: 11%

Goat Cheese Nuggets

MAKES: 16 nuggets | **PREP TIME:** 20 minutes, plus chilling time

Slightly tangy and velvety smooth, goat cheese is unlike any other cheese. In this recipe, it's blended with sun-dried tomatoes to create a creamy combination that will be turned into bite-size nuggets once chilled. The finishing touch of the ground walnuts adds a subtle sweet and nutty flavor that complements the mixture. These nuggets are also tasty when rolled in crushed pecans.

8 ounces goat cheese

3 oil-packed sun-dried tomatoes

1 teaspoon coconut oil

Pinch red pepper flakes

½ cup walnuts, coarsely ground

1. Put the goat cheese, sun-dried tomatoes, oil, and red pepper flakes in a blender. Blend until well combined. Transfer to a small bowl. Refrigerate until the mixture is firm enough to roll into balls.

2. Roll the goat cheese mixture into 16 small balls.

3. Roll the balls in the ground walnuts until they are completely coated. Store in the refrigerator in a sealed container for up to 1 week.

■ **VARIATION TIP:** The walnuts can be swapped out for pistachios for a more savory bite.

PER SERVING (1 NUGGET): Calories: 65; Fat: 6g; Protein: 3g; Total carbs: 1g; Fiber: 0g; Net carbs: 1g

MACROS: Fat: 75%; Protein: 21%; Carbs: 4%

Sriracha-Artichoke Bites

SERVES: 12 | **PREP TIME:** 15 minutes | **COOK TIME:** 35 minutes

This recipe is a two-for-one! It contains recipes for a spicy artichoke dip and a delicious cracker to scoop it up. However, you can use your favorite keto cracker recipe to pair with the dip. The cool sour cream and mayonnaise are contrasted with a spicy kick of Sriracha, but balanced out with the mild nutty flavor of artichoke.

FOR THE SCOOPS

Oil or nonstick cooking spray, for greasing
1½ cups grated mozzarella cheese
2 ounces (4 tablespoons) cream cheese
½ cup almond flour
2 tablespoons flaxseed meal
¼ teaspoon kosher salt

FOR THE ARTICHOKE DIP

Oil or nonstick cooking spray, for greasing
1 (14-ounce) can water-packed artichoke hearts, drained, rinsed, and chopped
½ cup sour cream
½ cup mayonnaise
1 tablespoon Sriracha
1 teaspoon garlic powder
¼ teaspoon kosher salt
½ cup grated Parmesan cheese
2 scallions, both white and green parts, chopped

TO MAKE THE SCOOPS

1. Preheat the oven to 350°F. Grease the back sides of 2 (24-cavity) mini muffin tins.

2. In a microwave-safe bowl, combine the mozzarella cheese and cream cheese. Microwave on high power in 20-second increments until melted and smooth.

3. Mix in the flour, flaxseed meal, and salt. Work into a ball of dough. (It will be greasy.)

4. Spread a sheet of parchment paper on the counter. Split the dough in two, and set one aside; place the other on the parchment paper. Place another sheet of parchment paper on top, and, with a rolling pin or the side of a drinking glass, roll the dough out very thin, $\frac{1}{16}$ to $\frac{1}{8}$ inch thick. (The thinner you roll them, the crunchier they'll be.) Repeat this step with the remaining half of the dough.

5. Using a 2¼-inch round cookie cutter or something similar, cut circles of dough. Set the muffin tins upside down, and place a circle of dough flat on top of each of the mounds.

6. Transfer the muffin tins to the oven, and bake, turning the tins about halfway through, for 10 to 15 minutes, or until the dough is completely golden brown. The dough will melt into a scoop. Remove from the oven. Let it cool for 1 minute, then gently pop off the scoops and cool completely. Store in an airtight container until ready to fill.

TO MAKE THE ARTICHOKE DIP

1. Preheat the oven to 350°F. Grease a small baking dish.

2. In a medium bowl, combine the artichoke hearts, sour cream, mayonnaise, Sriracha, garlic powder, and salt. Pour into the prepared baking dish, and cover loosely with aluminum foil.

3. Transfer the baking dish to the oven, and bake for 20 minutes. Remove from the oven. When cool enough to handle, spoon the mixture into the scoops.

4. Sprinkle with the cheese, garnish with the scallions, and serve.

PER SERVING (4 BITES): Calories: 203; Fat: 17g; Protein: 7g; Total carbs: 6g; Fiber: 3g; Net carbs: 3g

MACROS: Fat: 75%; Protein: 13%; Carbs: 12%

Marinated Feta and Artichokes

SERVES: 12 | **PREP TIME:** 10 minutes | **COOK TIME:** 2 hours

This recipe is simple to throw together, since it only requires combining ingredients and allowing the flavors to marinate in the oven. In my experience, the longer it marinates, the better! The creamy feta and artichoke pieces are soaked in fresh herbs and olive oil to provide a delicious bite and elevate your dining experience.

4 ounces feta, cut into ¼-inch cubes

4 ounces drained artichoke hearts, quartered lengthwise

1 pound Spanish olives with pits

1 cup almonds, preferably marcona

¾ cup extra-virgin olive oil

1 orange, peeled and very thinly sliced

½ fennel bulb, cored and thinly sliced

1 small red onion, thinly sliced

1 rosemary sprig

Pinch red pepper flakes

2 tablespoons red wine vinegar

1. Preheat the oven to 300°F.

2. In a shallow baking dish, toss together the feta, artichoke hearts, olives, almonds, oil, orange, fennel, onion, rosemary, red pepper flakes, and vinegar. Cover with aluminum foil.

3. Transfer the baking dish to the oven, and bake for 1½ hours.

4. Remove the foil. Bake for 20 to 30 more minutes. Remove from the oven. Let the mixture cool to room temperature before serving.

■ VARIATION TIP: The feta cheese can be replaced with mozzarella balls for a slightly different taste.

PER SERVING: Calories: 284; Fat: 27; Protein: 5g; Total carbs: 8g; Fiber: 4g; Net carbs: 4g

MACROS: Fat: 82%; Protein: 7%; Carbs: 11%

Chocolate-Almond Fat Bombs

DAIRY-FREE

VEGAN

MAKES: 12 fat bombs | **PREP TIME:** 5 minutes, plus time for the chocolate to set | **COOK TIME:** 5 minutes

Fat bombs are a bite-size snack, either savory or sweet, that packs a hefty amount of fat in order to help you meet your daily macros. This one combines the sweet and nutty flavors of chocolate and almonds. They can serve as a dessert at any event.

¾ cup coconut oil

6 tablespoons cocoa powder

2 tablespoons powdered erythritol

½ teaspoon vanilla extract

24 whole raw almonds

Coarse sea salt

1. Put 12 candy molds or mini muffin tin liners on a large sheet pan.

2. In a small saucepan, melt the oil over medium heat. Add the cocoa powder, erythritol, and vanilla. Whisk well to combine. Remove from the heat.

3. Spoon the mixture into the candy molds. Drop 2 almonds into each mold. Sprinkle sea salt on top of each. Refrigerate until the chocolate has set.

4. Remove the fat bombs from the molds, and store in a zip-top bag in the refrigerator for up to 1 week or in the freezer for up to 3 months.

■ **INGREDIENT TIP:** If you do not have powdered erythritol, you can put granulated erythritol into a coffee grinder to achieve the same results.

■ **VARIATION TIP:** Add chopped peanuts or shredded coconut in place of the almonds, and it'll be like a nice box of chocolates for your guests to choose from!

PER SERVING (1 FAT BOMB): Calories: 146; Fat: 15g; Protein: 1g; Total carbs: 4g; Fiber: 1g; Net carbs: 1g;

MACROS: Fat: 95%; Protein: 2%; Carbs: 3%

Taste-of-the-Mediterranean Fat Bombs

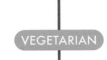

Olives are a key ingredient in Mediterranean cuisine. They also happen to be great for keto due to the generous portion of healthy fats they contain. These fat bombs also incorporate goat cheese and pesto for extra flair and flavor. Serve these chilled, and let them transport everyone to their favorite Mediterranean destination.

1 cup crumbled goat cheese
¼ cup jarred pesto
12 pitted Kalamata olives, finely chopped

½ cup finely chopped walnuts
1 tablespoon chopped fresh rosemary leaves

1. In a medium bowl, combine the goat cheese, pesto, and olives. Use a fork to mix well. Refrigerate for at least 4 hours to harden.

2. Using your hands, form the mixture into 6 balls about ¾ inch in diameter. The mixture will be sticky.

3. In a small bowl, combine the walnuts and rosemary.

4. Roll the goat cheese balls in the nut mixture to coat. Store in the refrigerator for up to 1 week or in the freezer for up to 1 month.

PER SERVING (1 FAT BOMB): Calories: 179; Fat: 17g; Protein: 6g; Total carbs: 2g; Fiber: 1g; Net carbs: 1g

MACROS: Fat: 82%; Protein: 13%; Carbs: 5%

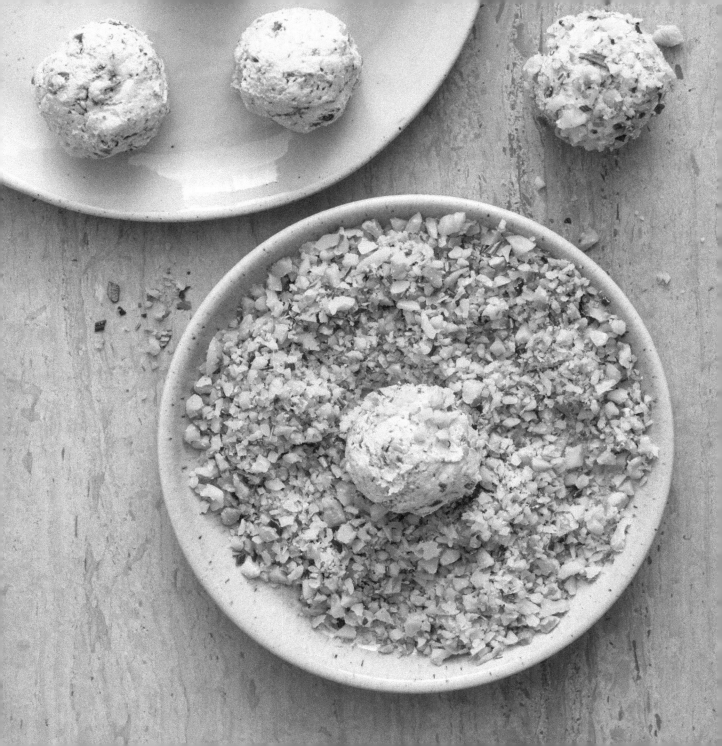

Bacon-Chive Fat Bombs

NUT-FREE

SERVES: 8 | **PREP TIME:** 5 minutes

There's something special about the combination of cheese and chives. I have yet to have a dish that contains those two ingredients and isn't delicious! Once you add bacon to this dynamic duo, you've simply created a masterpiece. These savory appetizers are quick and easy to make. Because of the high fat content, your guests are sure to be satisfied quickly.

8 ounces full-fat cream cheese, at room temperature
4 tablespoons (½ stick) butter, at room temperature

4 bacon slices, cooked, cooled, and crumbled
1 tablespoon minced fresh chives
¼ teaspoon freshly ground black pepper
¼ cup grated Parmesan cheese

1. In a bowl, combine the cream cheese, butter, bacon, chives, and pepper.

2. Divide the mixture into 8 small balls.

3. Roll the balls in the Parmesan cheese to coat them lightly. Refrigerate until ready to serve.

PER SERVING (1 FAT BOMB): Calories: 183; Fat: 18g; Protein: 4g; Total carbs: 2g; Fiber: 0g; Net carbs: 2g

MACROS: Fat: 87%; Protein: 10%; Carbs: 3%

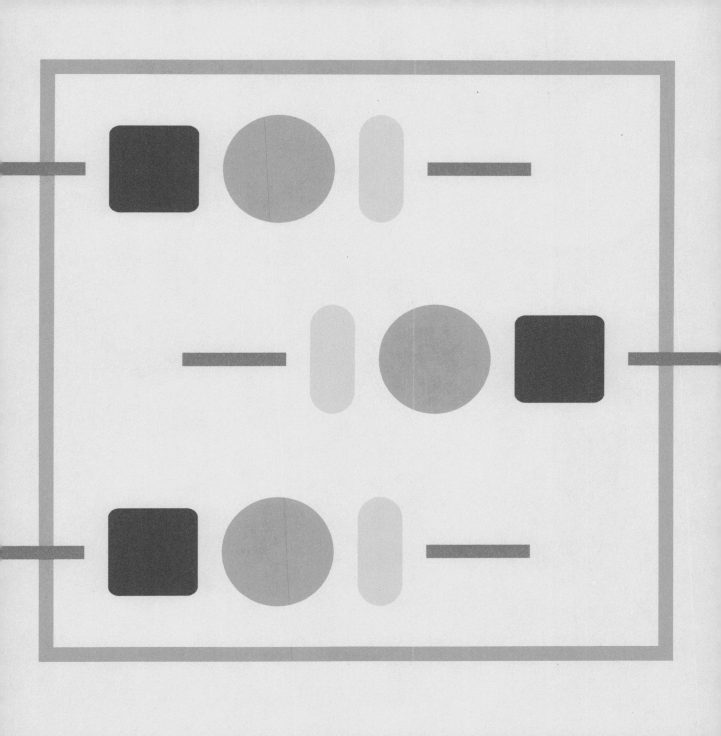

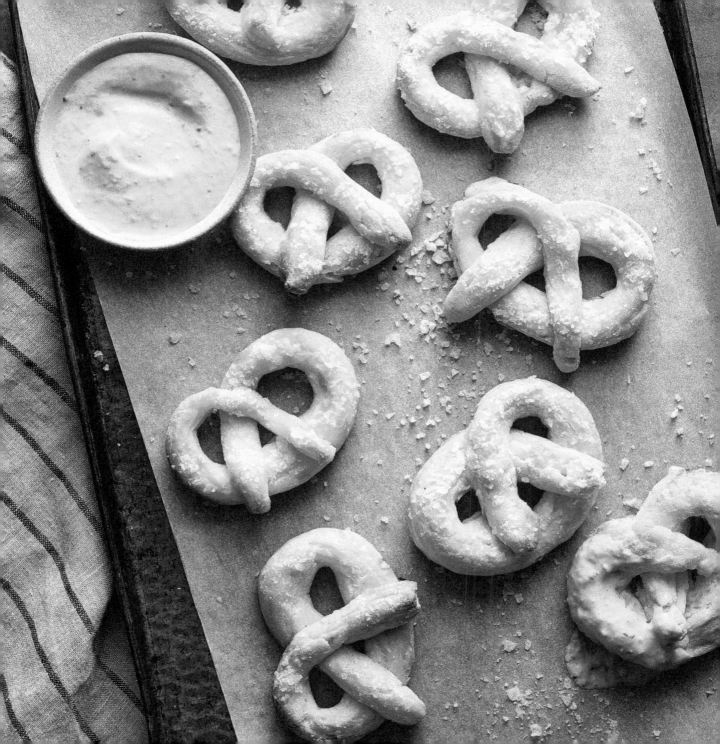

CHAPTER 4

Breads and Crackers

Almond-Flour Crackers

SERVES: 6 | **PREP TIME:** 10 minutes | **COOK TIME:** 25 minutes

Who doesn't love a good cracker? Crackers tend to be sturdier than chips but lighter and crispier than bread. They're the ideal vessel for all your appetizer needs. Top these crispy crackers with sliced meats and cheeses for a phenomenal charcuterie bite, or dunk them into your favorite dip for a delicious treat.

1 cup blanched almond flour
¼ cup powdered Parmesan cheese
¼ cup water

½ teaspoon garlic powder
½ teaspoon Italian seasoning
Coarse sea salt

1. Preheat the oven to 350°F.

2. In a medium bowl, combine the flour, cheese, water, garlic powder, and Italian seasoning. Stir to form a dough.

3. Place the dough between 2 pieces of parchment paper. Using a rolling pin or wine bottle, roll the dough into a thin rectangle slightly smaller than your sheet pan.

4. Remove the top piece of parchment paper. Lift the bottom piece of parchment paper to transfer the dough to a sheet pan.

5. Lightly sprinkle salt over the dough, and gently press it in.

6. Using a pizza wheel or sharp knife, cut the dough into 1-by-2-inch crackers, or any desired size.

Continued ›››

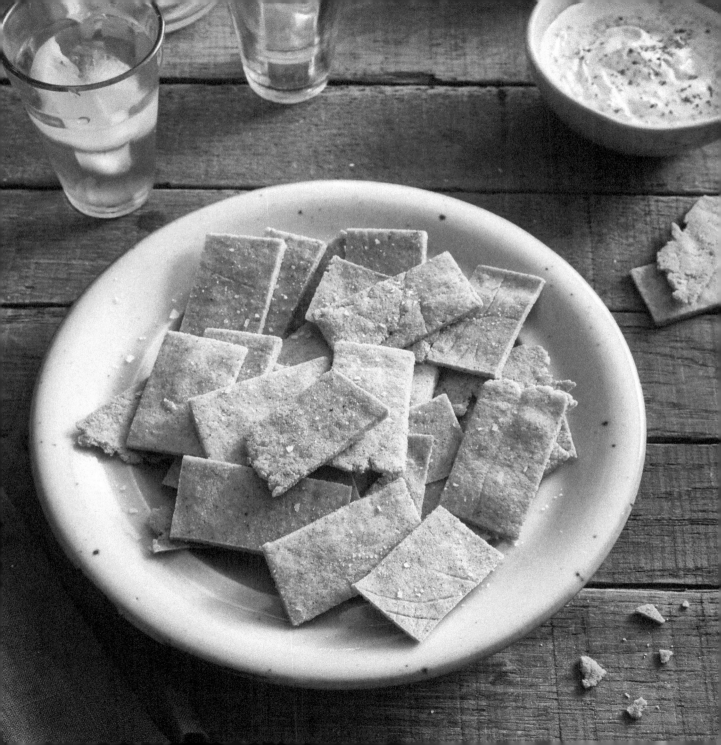

Almond-Flour Crackers *continued*

7. Using a toothpick, create a small hole in the center of each cracker.

8. Transfer the sheet pan to the oven, and bake for about 25 minutes, or until the crackers have lightly browned. Remove from the oven. Let cool on a wire rack, then break the crackers apart. Store for up to 1 week in a zip-top bag in the pantry.

■ INGREDIENT TIP: Be sure to use finely milled almond flour and not almond meal in order to get the best results.

PER SERVING: Calories: 110; Fat: 9g; Protein: 4g; Total carbs: 4g; Fiber: 2g; Net carbs: 2g

MACROS: Fat: 70%; Protein: 15%; Carbs: 15%

Cheddar-Chive Biscuits

MAKES: 10 biscuits | **PREP TIME:** 10 minutes | **COOK TIME:** 20 minutes

These soft, fluffy, low-carb biscuits are absolutely divine. Serve these warm with plenty of butter for topping. The flavors of cheddar and chive create an exquisite combination of salty and savory that will surely leave your guests hoping for more!

1¾ cups finely milled almond flour

2 tablespoons coconut flour

1 tablespoon baking powder

¼ teaspoon sea salt

½ cup sour cream

½ cup shredded sharp cheddar cheese

4 tablespoons (¼ stick) unsalted butter, melted, plus more for serving

2 large eggs, at room temperature

2 tablespoons finely chopped fresh chives

2 tablespoons grated Parmesan cheese

1. Preheat the oven to 375°F. Line a large sheet pan with parchment paper or a silicone baking mat.

2. To make the dough, in a large bowl sift together the almond flour, coconut flour, baking powder, and salt. Add the sour cream, cheddar cheese, butter, eggs, and chives. Using a fork, combine until fully incorporated.

3. Drop the dough by large spoonfuls onto the prepared sheet pan, and sprinkle the top of each biscuit with the Parmesan cheese. Transfer the sheet pan to the oven, and bake for 20 minutes, or until the biscuits are lightly golden brown on top.

4. Serve your biscuits hot from the oven with butter. Store any leftovers in the refrigerator for up to 5 days, or freeze for up to 3 weeks.

■ **VARIATION TIP:** Experiment with different types of cheese for different flavors.

PER SERVING (1 BISCUIT): Calories: 202; Fat: 18g; Protein: 7g; Total carbs: 5g; Fiber: 2g; Net carbs: 3g

MACROS: Fat: 78%; Protein: 13%; Carbs: 9%

Soft-Baked Pretzels with Spicy Mustard Dip

SERVES: 10 | **PREP TIME:** 20 minutes, plus 40 minutes to proof and rise
COOK TIME: 25 to 30 minutes, plus cooling time

You can always find pretzels at various games, carnivals, and concerts. They are clearly a crowd favorite! These keto-friendly pretzels can be molded into a classic pretzel shape, as shown on page 64, or shaped into simple sticks, perfect for dipping and passing around a group of friends. The mustard dip takes this appetizer to the next level with a spicy kick to keep you on your toes.

FOR THE SPICY MUSTARD DIP

¼ cup full-fat mayonnaise
¼ cup prepared yellow mustard
1½ teaspoons prepared horseradish
1 teaspoon Tabasco sauce
½ teaspoon sea salt
½ teaspoon onion powder
¼ teaspoon red pepper flakes
¼ teaspoon freshly ground
    black pepper
¼ teaspoon garlic powder

FOR THE PRETZELS

1 tablespoon yeast
1 teaspoon inulin fiber or sugar
3 tablespoons warm water
2 cups shredded part-skim mozzarella
    cheese, melted
2 tablespoons cream cheese, at room
    temperature
¾ cup coconut flour
2 teaspoons baking powder
¼ teaspoon xanthan gum
2 large eggs, at room temperature
1 large egg white, at room temperature
Coarse sea salt

TO MAKE THE SPICY MUSTARD DIP

1. In a medium bowl, combine the mayonnaise, mustard, horseradish, Tabasco, salt, onion powder, red pepper flakes, black pepper, and garlic powder. Cover, and refrigerate for at least 30 minutes to allow the flavors to develop. Store any left-over mustard sauce in the refrigerator for up to 5 days.

TO MAKE THE PRETZELS

1. Proof the yeast: Put the yeast and inulin fiber in a small bowl large enough to allow the yeast to expand.

2. Add the warm water, and stir. Cover the bowl with a kitchen towel, and let rest for 10 minutes. The yeast has properly proofed when it expands and bubbles.

3. While the yeast is proofing, line a large sheet pan with a silicone baking mat or parchment paper.

4. Put the mozzarella cheese in a large, microwave-safe bowl. Microwave on high power in 30-second increments, making sure to stir each time, until fully melted.

5. Add the cream cheese to the melted mozzarella cheese, and mix until combined.

6. Using a rubber spatula, stir in the flour, baking powder, and xanthan gum.

7. Add the eggs and proofed yeast. Combine well until a dough comes together.

8. Using wet hands, lightly knead the dough. Divide into 10 equal balls, being sure to keep your hands wet so the dough doesn't stick. Roll each ball between your hands to form a pretzel stick about ¾ inch thick. (If you're feeling fancy, form into a classic pretzel shape!)

9. Put the pretzels on the prepared sheet pan. Using your hands, smooth any cracks on the surface or sides of the pretzels.

Continued ›››

10. In a small bowl, beat the egg white with a whisk until foamy. Use a pastry brush to brush the egg onto the pretzels. Let rest and slightly rise in a warm, draft-free place for 30 minutes.

11. While the pretzels are rising, preheat the oven to 375°F.

12. Sprinkle the pretzels with coarse sea salt.

13. Transfer the sheet pan to the oven, and bake for 25 to 30 minutes, or until the pretzels are golden brown. Remove from the oven. Let them cool for 2 to 3 minutes in the pan, then transfer them to a wire rack to cool fully. Store any leftover pretzels in the refrigerator for up to 5 days, or freeze for up to 3 weeks.

■ **VARIATION TIP:** The dough for this recipe is very flexible, so you can get creative with any shape of pretzel you like!

PER SERVING (1 PRETZEL WITH DIP): Calories: 144; Fat: 11g; Protein: 8g; Total carbs: 3g; Fiber: 1g; Net carbs: 2g

---

MACROS: Fat: 69%; Protein: 24%; Carbs: 7%

Sour Cream "Corn" Bread

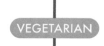

VEGETARIAN

SERVES: 9 | **PREP TIME:** 10 minutes | **COOK TIME:** 30 minutes

Corn bread is a Southern comfort food classic. It's a great addition to any bread-basket. Needless to say, there's no corn in this recipe. However, that slightly sweet and nutty taste found in corn bread is achieved by using coconut flour. Furthermore, the addition of sour cream makes this "corn" bread super moist and delectable.

5 tablespoons unsalted butter, melted, plus more for the pan
1 cup almond flour
2½ tablespoons coconut flour
2½ teaspoons baking powder

1 teaspoon monk fruit/erythritol blend sweetener
½ teaspoon sea salt
¼ teaspoon baking soda
5 large eggs
2 tablespoons sour cream

1. Preheat the oven to 350°F. Thoroughly coat an 8-by-8-inch baking pan with butter.

2. In a medium bowl, stir together the almond flour, coconut flour, baking powder, sweetener, salt, and baking soda. Using an electric hand mixer on medium speed, mix in the eggs and sour cream until well combined. Stir in the melted butter. Pour the batter into the prepared pan.

3. Transfer the baking pan to the oven, and bake for 25 to 30 minutes, or until the bread is golden brown and a toothpick inserted into the center comes out clean.

4. Cut the bread into 9 squares, and serve warm.

PER SERVING (1 SQUARE): Calories: 166; Fat: 15g; Protein: 6g; Total carbs: 3g; Fiber: 1g; Net carbs: 2g

MACROS: Fat: 79%; Protein: 14%; Carbs: 7%

Keto Bagels

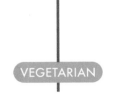

SERVES: 8 | **PREP TIME:** 15 minutes | **COOK TIME:** 20 minutes

How do you enjoy your bagels? With cream cheese and lox? Peanut butter and jelly? Avocado and sea salt? These aren't your traditional gluten-filled bagels, but they will surely pair perfectly with any topping. You can even set up a bagel bar and offer various fruits, vegetables, meats, cheese, and spreads for your guests to create their own personalized experiences.

1½ cups finely milled almond flour
1 tablespoon coconut flour
1 tablespoon baking powder
½ teaspoon kosher salt
½ teaspoon xanthan gum (optional)

2 large eggs
2 cups shredded part-skim mozzarella cheese
2 ounces full-fat cream cheese
2 tablespoons sesame seeds (optional)

1. Preheat the oven to 350°F. Line a large sheet pan with parchment paper.

2. In a large bowl, whisk together the almond flour, coconut flour, baking powder, salt, and xanthan gum (if using).

3. In a small bowl, beat the eggs to combine. Measure out 2 tablespoons, and set aside.

4. In a microwave-safe bowl, combine the mozzarella cheese and cream cheese. Microwave on high power, stirring halfway through, for 1½ minutes, or until the cheese looks smooth when stirred.

5. Add the flour mixture and remaining beaten eggs. Stir until well combined.

6. Divide the dough into 8 portions. Roll each portion into a ball, and press a thumb in the center of each ball, making the hole in the bagel. Stretch the bagel to open it up a bit more.

7. Place the bagels on the prepared sheet pan, and brush the tops of the bagels with the reserved 2 tablespoons of beaten egg.

8. Sprinkle with the sesame seeds (if using).

9. Transfer the sheet pan to the oven, and bake for 15 minutes, or until the bagels have lightly browned. Remove from the oven. Store in an airtight container in the refrigerator for up to 1 week or in the freezer for up to 3 months.

■ **VARIATION TIP:** Choose a variety of toppings to place on your bagels and transform them. Try shredded cheddar, poppy seeds, or even cinnamon for a fun twist.

PER SERVING (1 BAGEL): Calories: 213; Fat: 17g; Protein: 13g; Total carbs: 5g; Fiber: 2g; Net carbs: 3g

MACROS: Fat: 67%; Protein: 23%; Carbs: 10%

Almond-Flour Bread

MAKES: 1 loaf (16 slices) | **PREP TIME:** 15 minutes | **COOK TIME:** 30 minutes, plus 10 minutes to cool

This bread is extremely versatile. You can slice it and serve it as toast, or top with favorites such as balsamic vinegar and chopped tomatoes for crispy bruschetta bites. The mixture of almond flour and protein powder creates a great texture, and the psyllium husk provides the chewiness that bread lovers everywhere crave.

Olive oil cooking spray
2 cups finely milled almond flour
¼ cup unflavored protein powder
2 tablespoons psyllium husk powder
2 teaspoons baking powder
1 teaspoon kosher salt

4 large eggs
3 tablespoons unsalted butter, melted
2 teaspoons granulated monk fruit sweetener
1 teaspoon apple cider vinegar
½ cup hot water

1. Preheat the oven to 350°F. Line the bottom and 2 long sides of a 9-by-5-inch loaf pan with parchment paper. Mist the paper with cooking spray.

2. In a large bowl, whisk together the flour, protein powder, psyllium husk powder, baking powder, and salt.

3. In a medium bowl, whisk together the eggs, butter, monk fruit sweetener, and vinegar.

4. To make the batter, add the egg mixture to the flour mixture, and stir to combine.

5. Add the hot water, and stir until completely combined.

6. Scrape the batter into the prepared loaf pan.

7. Transfer the loaf pan to the oven, and bake for 30 minutes, or until a toothpick inserted into the center of the loaf comes out clean. Remove from the oven. Let cool for 10 minutes in the pan before cutting. Store in an airtight bag in the refrigerator for up to 1 week or in the freezer for up to 3 months.

PER SERVING (1 SLICE): Calories: 119; Fat: 9g; Protein: 6g; Total carbs: 4g; Fiber: 2g; Net carbs: 2g

MACROS: Fat: 67%; Protein: 20%; Carbs: 13%

Onion-Garlic Pita-Style Bread VEGETARIAN

MAKES: 6 pitas | **PREP TIME:** 15 minutes | **COOK TIME:** 25 to 35 minutes, plus cooling time

This pita-style bread recipe is full of flavor. The onion and garlic powders lend savory notes to each bite. Although you won't be able to get the infamous pita "pocket," you can surely pile on your favorite fillings or fold it in half like a sandwich. It's also great for dipping!

3 tablespoons golden flaxseed meal

3 cups finely milled almond flour, sifted

1 tablespoon psyllium husk powder

2 teaspoons sesame seeds

2 teaspoons baking powder

½ teaspoon xanthan gum

½ teaspoon sea salt

½ teaspoon onion powder

½ teaspoon garlic powder

1 cup hot water

1 tablespoon extra-virgin olive oil or melted coconut oil

2 large eggs, at room temperature

1 tablespoon salted butter, melted

¼ cup chopped fresh parsley

Sea salt flakes

1. Preheat the oven to 400°F. Line a large sheet pan with a silicone baking mat or parchment paper.

2. Put the flaxseed meal in a coffee grinder, and grind it into a fine powder.

3. In a large bowl, combine the flaxseed-meal powder, almond flour, psyllium husk powder, sesame seeds, baking powder, xanthan gum, salt, onion powder, and garlic powder.

4. Add the hot water, oil, and eggs. Using a silicone spatula, mix well to form a dough.

5. Scoop 6 equal portions of the dough onto the prepared sheet pan. Using wet hands, form into circles. Be sure to keep your hands wet because the dough will be very sticky.

6. Use a pastry brush to brush each pita with the butter.

7. Sprinkle the tops of the pitas evenly with the parsley and sea salt flakes.

8. Transfer the sheet pan to the oven, and bake for 25 to 35 minutes, or until the pitas have lightly browned. Remove from the oven. Let cool fully on the sheet pan before serving. Store any leftovers in the refrigerator for up to 5 days, or freeze for up to 3 weeks.

■ **PREP TIP:** Be careful not to overbake the pita once it's lightly browned, or it will lose its flexibility.

PER SERVING (1 PITA): Calories: 363; Fat: 32g; Protein: 13g; Total carbs: 13g; Fiber: 7g; Net carbs: 6g

MACROS: Fat: 73%; Protein: 13%; Carbs: 14%

Spicy Cheddar Wafers

MAKES: 30 wafers | **PREP TIME:** 10 minutes, plus 2 hours to chill | **COOK TIME:** 25 minutes

These cheddar wafers are bursting with flavor. This recipe calls for various savory seasonings and even cayenne to lend a subtle spicy note. The almond and coconut flours make the wafers sturdier and closer to cracker form. They are good enough to enjoy alone or alongside your favorite dip.

1 cup almond flour
2 tablespoons coconut flour
¼ teaspoon kosher salt
¼ teaspoon cayenne
¼ teaspoon garlic powder
¼ teaspoon onion powder

5 tablespoons unsalted butter, at room temperature
1 ounce cream cheese, at room temperature
4 ounces sharp cheddar cheese, shredded
¼ cup finely chopped pecans

1. In a small bowl, stir together the almond flour, coconut flour, salt, cayenne, garlic powder, and onion powder.

2. In a large bowl, use an electric hand mixer on medium speed to cream together the butter and cream cheese.

3. Add the cheddar cheese, and mix until well combined.

4. Add the almond flour mixture, and mix to combine.

5. Stir in the pecans.

6. Place the dough on plastic wrap or parchment paper, and form into a log about 2½ inches thick. Wrap the dough tightly, and refrigerate for at least 2 hours, or until firm.

7. Preheat the oven to 300°F. Line a sheet pan with parchment paper.

8. Cut the chilled dough into ¼-inch-thick slices, and place on the prepared sheet pan.

9. Transfer the sheet pan to the oven, and bake for 20 to 25 minutes, or until the wafers are lightly golden brown. Remove from the oven. Let cool completely on the pan before removing.

■ PREP TIP: The dough for these cheddar wafers can be kept in the freezer or refrigerated until needed, saving you lots of time on the day of your event.

PER SERVING (3 WAFERS): Calories: 185; Fat: 18g; Protein: 5g; Total carbs: 3g; Fiber: 2g; Net carbs: 1g

MACROS: Fat: 83%; Protein: 11%; Carbs: 6%

Orange, Olive Oil, and Poppy Seed Muffins

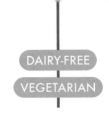

MAKES: 9 muffins | **PREP TIME:** 15 minutes | **COOK TIME:** 20 minutes, plus cooling time

These muffins have a slightly sweet and fruity flavor perfect for brunch or dessert. You'll only be using orange zest, so you don't have to worry about increased sugar. However, the zest is enough to get the orange flavor to shine through!

4 large eggs

1 large egg yolk

1 cup almond flour

6 tablespoons monk fruit/erythritol blend sweetener

⅓ cup olive oil

¼ cup coconut flour

2½ teaspoons baking powder

2 teaspoons grated orange zest

2 teaspoons poppy seeds

1 teaspoon vanilla extract

¼ teaspoon kosher salt

1. Preheat the oven to 350°F. Line a standard muffin tin with 9 liners.

2. In the bowl of a stand mixer fitted with the whisk attachment, or in a large bowl and using an electric hand mixer, whip the eggs and egg yolk on medium speed for about 2 minutes, or until light and foamy.

3. Add the remaining ingredients. Mix on medium speed until well combined, stopping to scrape down the sides of the bowl at least once.

4. Evenly divide the batter among the muffin cups. Bake for 15 to 20 minutes, or until the muffins are golden brown on top. Let them cool in the pan for 10 minutes, then transfer to a wire rack to fully cool. Store at room temperature in an airtight container for up to 3 days, or freeze for up to 1 month.

PER SERVING (1 MUFFIN): Calories: 215; Fat: 17g; Protein: 6g; Total carbs: 12g; Fiber: 2g; Net carbs: 2g

MACROS: Fat: 80%; Protein: 12%; Carbs: 8%

Pepperoni-Parmesan Chips

NUT-FREE

SERVES: 6 | **PREP TIME:** 5 minutes | **COOK TIME:** 15 minutes

Nothing screams pizza like pepperoni. It's a universal favorite. When baked, pepperoni slices turn into the perfect chips, and the addition of Parmesan takes them to the next level. They have the saltiness and crispness that everyone looks for in a chip. Dip them into marinara for intense pizza flavor, or try any of your favorite dips.

1 (6-ounce) bag sliced pepperoni
½ cup finely grated Parmesan cheese

1. Preheat the oven to 425°F. Line a sheet pan with parchment paper.

2. Lay each pepperoni slice down on the parchment paper, trying not to overlap.

3. Transfer the sheet pan to the oven, and bake for 10 minutes. Remove from the oven, and leave the oven on.

4. Dot each pepperoni slice with a paper towel to soak up the grease. Immediately shake enough cheese over all the pepperoni slices to lightly cover them.

5. Return the sheet pan to the oven, and bake for 3 to 4 minutes, or until the pepperoni slices look crispy. Remove from the oven. Transfer the slices to paper towels. Store leftovers in an airtight bag for up to 2 days in the refrigerator. Reheat in the oven to bring back their crispness.

PER SERVING: Calories: 175; Fat: 15g; Protein: 9g; Total carbs: 1g; Fiber: 0g; Net carbs: 1g

MACROS: Fat: 76%; Protein: 22%; Carbs: 2%

Garlic Breadsticks

MAKES: 8 breadsticks | **PREP TIME:** 15 minutes, plus 30 minutes to rest | **COOK TIME:** 15 minutes

These garlic breadsticks are insanely flavorful! Breadsticks are usually served alongside your favorite Italian dish or right next to a big leafy salad. However, turn these breadsticks into an even more ideal appetizer by cutting them into smaller pieces and creating garlic bread bites. Your guests can dunk them into various sauces, like marinara or alfredo, for wildly unique experiences.

1 cup almond flour
2 tablespoons coconut flour
2 teaspoons baking powder
1 teaspoon garlic powder
¼ teaspoon kosher salt

2½ cups grated mozzarella cheese
½ cup grated sharp cheddar cheese
2 ounces (4 tablespoons) cream cheese
2 large eggs
2 tablespoons garlic salt

1. Preheat the oven to 400°F. Line a sheet pan with parchment paper.

2. In a small bowl, combine the almond flour, coconut flour, baking powder, garlic powder, and salt.

3. In a medium microwave-safe bowl, combine the mozzarella cheese, cheddar cheese, and cream cheese. Microwave on high speed in 30-second increments until the mixture is melted and smooth. Remove from the microwave. Stir to blend.

4. To make the dough, stir in half of the flour mixture. Add the eggs and remaining flour mixture. Mix together until incorporated. Let the dough rest for 30 minutes to make it easier to work with.

5. Spread a piece of parchment paper on the counter. Using damp hands, make a ball out of the dough, and split it in half. Place one half on the parchment paper on the counter, and split into 4 equal parts. Flatten each part, then with your palms, roll each part into a 6- to 8-inch breadstick. Put the 4 breadsticks on the prepared sheet pan. Repeat with the remaining dough to make 8 breadsticks total.

6. Sprinkle the garlic salt over the breadsticks.

7. Transfer the sheet pan to the oven and bake, turning halfway through, for 13 to 15 minutes, or until the breadsticks are golden brown. Remove from the oven. Serve.

■ **PREP TIP:** Keep some water nearby to keep your hands damp so the dough is easier to work with.

PER SERVING (1 BREADSTICK): Calories: 272; Fat: 22g; Protein: 14g; Total carbs: 6g; Fiber: 2g; Net carbs: 4g

MACROS: Fat: 70%; Protein: 22%; Carbs: 8%

Flaxseed-Meal Tortillas

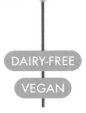

DAIRY-FREE

VEGAN

MAKES: 8 tortillas | **PREP TIME:** 10 minutes, plus 10 minutes to rest | **COOK TIME:** 10 minutes

A taco bar is a festive addition to any party or gathering. But what is a taco bar without tortillas? Luckily, these flaxseed-meal tortillas are a great stand-in for your traditional flour tortillas. The flaxseed meal is mild and unnoticeable. Pile these tortillas high with your favorite fillings, fold, and enjoy!

¾ cup golden flaxseed meal
¼ cup coconut flour
1 tablespoon psyllium husk powder
½ teaspoon xanthan gum

½ teaspoon sea salt
1 cup hot water
1 tablespoon coconut or olive oil

1. Put the flaxseed meal in a coffee grinder, and grind into a fine powder. In a large bowl, combine the powder, flour, psyllium husk powder, xanthan gum, and salt.

2. Add the hot water and oil. Using a silicone spatula, mix well to form a dough. Cover with a kitchen towel, and let rest for about 10 minutes.

3. Using your hands, form the dough into 8 equal balls. Flatten each ball between 2 sheets of parchment paper, or use a tortilla press, to form 8 (5-inch) tortillas.

4. In a large nonstick skillet, cook each tortilla over medium heat for about 10 to 15 seconds and then flip. Cook for 20 to 30 seconds total, or until both sides are golden. Keep the tortillas warm by wrapping them in a kitchen towel. Serve immediately. Store any leftovers in the refrigerator for up to 5 days, or freeze for up to 3 weeks. To warm, simply reheat in the skillet until just warm.

■ **VARIATION TIP:** Add various spices, such as onion and garlic powder, for extra flavor.

PER SERVING (1 TORTILLA): Calories: 80; Fat: 7g; Protein: 2g; Total carbs: 3g; Fiber: 3g; Net carbs: 0g

MACROS: Fat: 74%; Protein: 9%; Carbs: 17%

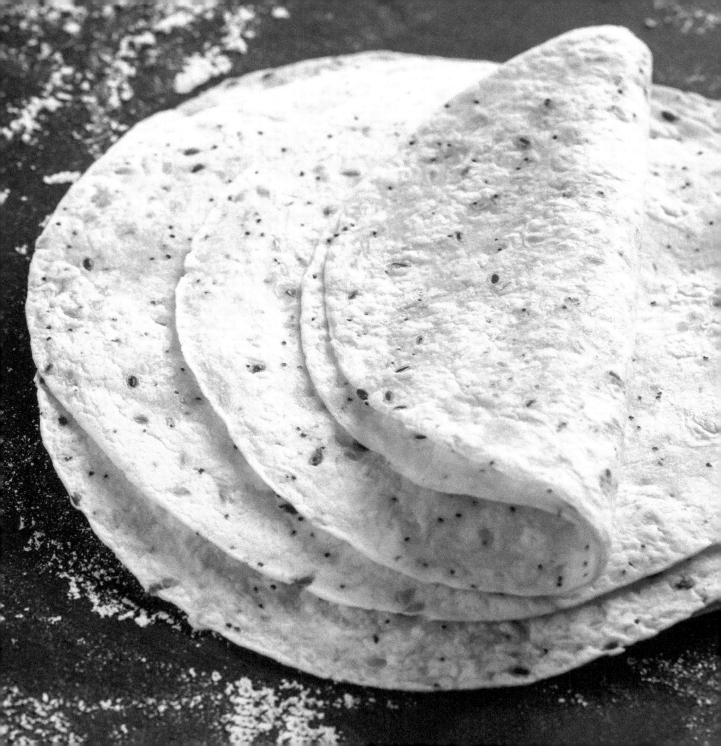

Savory Naan

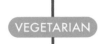

MAKES: 6 naan | **PREP TIME:** 15 minutes | **COOK TIME:** 15 to 20 minutes, plus cooling time

This savory naan recipe is tasty and extremely versatile. It makes well-seasoned dough that forms the best pillowy-soft, low-carb naan. Use this naan to scoop up delicious hummus or spicy curry, or slather it with salted butter. Regardless of the pairing, this naan will prove to be the perfect vessel.

1½ tablespoons golden flaxseed meal
1½ cups finely milled almond flour, sifted
2 teaspoons psyllium husk powder
2 teaspoons sesame seeds
2 teaspoons baking powder
½ teaspoon onion powder
½ teaspoon garlic powder
¼ teaspoon xanthan gum

¼ teaspoon sea salt
1 cup hot water
1 teaspoon extra-virgin olive oil
2 large eggs, at room temperature
1 tablespoon salted butter, melted
2 tablespoons fresh flat-leaf parsley, chopped
2 teaspoons sea salt flakes

1. Preheat the oven to 375°F. Line a large sheet pan with a silicone baking mat or parchment paper.

2. Put the flaxseed meal in a coffee grinder, and grind into a fine powder.

3. In a large bowl, combine the flaxseed meal powder, almond flour, psyllium husk powder, sesame seeds, baking powder, onion powder, garlic powder, xanthan gum, and salt.

4. Add the hot water, oil, and eggs. Using a silicone spatula, mix well to form a dough.

5. Scoop 6 equal portions of the dough onto the prepared sheet pan. Using wet hands, form into circles. Be sure to keep your hands wet because the dough will be very sticky.

6. Use a pastry brush to brush each naan with the butter.

7. Sprinkle the tops of the naans evenly with the parsley and sea salt flakes.

8. Transfer the sheet pan to the oven, and bake for 15 to 20 minutes, or until the naans have lightly browned. Remove from the oven. Let cool slightly on the sheet pan before serving. Store any leftovers in the refrigerator for up to 5 days, or freeze for up to 3 weeks.

■ VARIATION TIP: If you're looking to make this recipe dairy-free, simply replace the butter with coconut oil.

PER SERVING (1 NAAN): Calories: 200; Fat: 17g; Protein: 8g; Total carbs: 6g; Fiber: 4g; Net carbs: 2g

MACROS: Fat: 73%; Protein: 14%; Carbs: 13%

Sesame Seed Crackers

MAKES: 20 crackers | **PREP TIME:** 15 minutes | **COOK TIME:** 50 minutes to 1 hour, plus cooling time

Crunchy, crispy, and cheesy, these sesame seed crackers tick all the boxes! This recipe is easy to put together. Have fun cutting them into different shapes and sizes—once the dough is rolled out, let your creativity take control. Your guests can enjoy these by the handful or paired with a delicious dip.

½ cup shredded sharp cheddar cheese

½ cup finely grated shelf-stable
   Parmesan cheese

½ cup grated Parmesan cheese

½ cup coconut flour

½ cup sesame seeds

2 teaspoons psyllium husk powder

1 teaspoon baking powder

1 teaspoon onion powder

1 teaspoon garlic powder

1 teaspoon dried basil

1 teaspoon dried oregano

½ teaspoon sea salt

¼ teaspoon freshly ground black pepper

¼ teaspoon red pepper flakes

1 cup water

3 tablespoons avocado oil or
   extra-virgin olive oil

1 large egg, at room temperature

2 tablespoons white sesame seeds,
   divided

2 tablespoons black sesame seeds,
   divided

1. Preheat the oven to 350°F. Line a large sheet pan with parchment paper.

2. In a large mixing bowl, combine the cheddar cheese, shelf-stable Parmesan cheese, grated Parmesan cheese, coconut flour, sesame seeds, psyllium husk powder, baking powder, onion powder, garlic powder, basil, oregano, salt, black pepper, and red pepper flakes. Stir until well combined.

3. Add the water, oil, and egg. Stir until a smooth dough forms.

4. Divide the dough in half, and roll one half out thinly between 2 sheets of parchment paper. The thinner you roll out the dough, the crispier the crackers.

5. Use a pizza cutter to cut the dough into crackers, and carefully place on the prepared sheet pan. (You may need to transfer them using a pancake spatula.)

6. Sprinkle 1 tablespoon of white sesame seeds and 1 tablespoon of black sesame seeds on top of the crackers.

7. Transfer the sheet pan to the oven, and bake for 25 to 30 minutes, or until the crackers have lightly browned around the edges. Remove from the oven. Repeat with the other half of the dough. Let the crackers cool fully on the sheet pan before serving. Store any leftovers in the refrigerator for up to 5 days, or freeze for up to 3 weeks.

PER SERVING (4 CRACKERS): Calories: 394; Fat: 35g; Protein: 15g; Total carbs: 8g; Fiber: 4g; Net carbs: 4g

MACROS: Fat: 77%; Protein: 15%; Carbs: 8%

Crispy Parmesan Crackers

NUT-FREE

MAKES: 8 crackers | **PREP TIME:** 10 minutes | **COOK TIME:** 5 minutes

When shredded or grated Parmesan cheese is melted, it creates these buttery, flavorful, lacy crackers that are simply irresistible! Since these crackers are quite dainty, they're not necessarily for dipping. However, they do serve as an amazing chip replacement. The salty crunch you crave is sure to be satisfied.

1 teaspoon unsalted butter
8 ounces full-fat Parmesan cheese, shredded or freshly grated

1. Preheat the oven to 400°F. Line a sheet pan with parchment paper. Lightly grease the paper with the butter.

2. Spoon the cheese in mounds, spread evenly apart, onto the prepared sheet pan. Use the back of a spoon to press the mounds until they are flat.

3. Transfer the sheet pan to the oven, and bake for about 5 minutes, or until the cracker edges have browned but the centers are still pale. Remove from the oven.

4. Use a spatula to move the crackers to paper towels. Lightly blot the tops with additional paper towels. Let cool completely. Store in a sealed container in the refrigerator for up to 4 days.

■ **INGREDIENT TIP:** Make sure the Parmesan cheese is freshly grated or shredded. Don't use the type in a canister because it won't melt properly.

PER SERVING (1 CRACKER): Calories: 123; Fat: 8g; Protein: 8g; Total carbs: 4g; Fiber: 0g; Net carbs: 4g

MACROS: Fat: 60%; Protein: 28%; Carbs: 12%

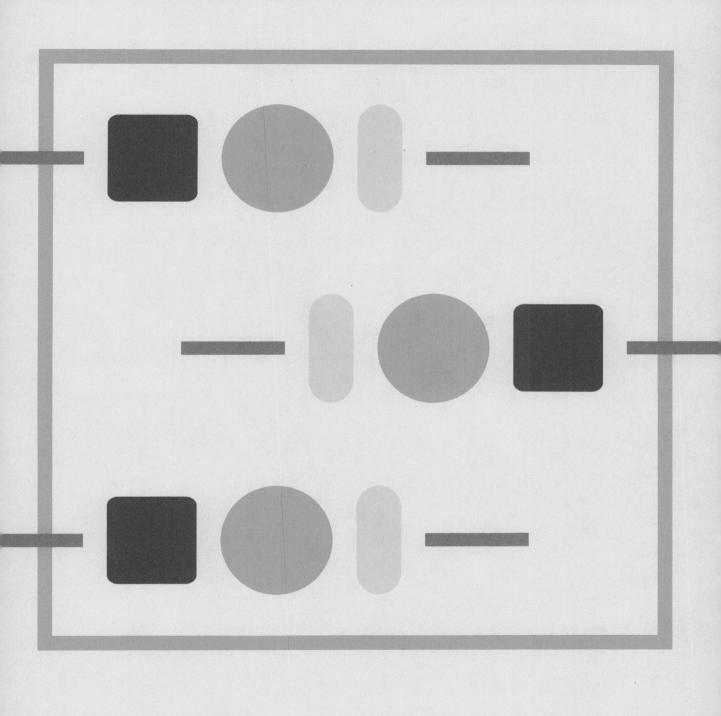

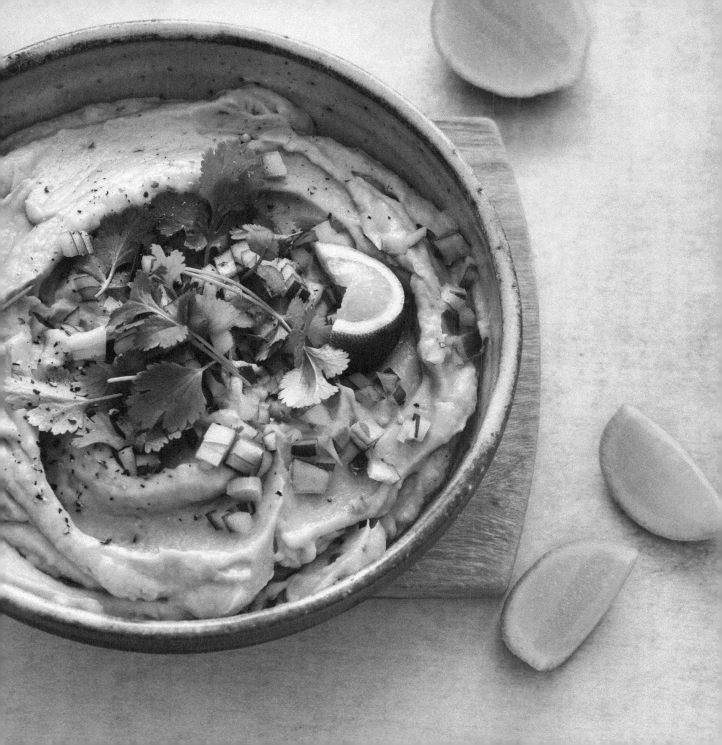

CHAPTER 5

Dips and Spreads

5-Minute Cheese Sauce

NUT-FREE

MAKES: 1 cup | **PREP TIME:** 5 minutes | **COOK TIME:** 5 minutes

The only thing better than a cheese sauce is a quick cheese sauce! This creamy, delicious recipe is easy to make, contains very few ingredients, and can jazz up any appetizer table. You can serve it alongside various vegetables or top up a plate of low-carb tortilla chips for some amazing nachos.

4 ounces cream cheese
½ cup heavy cream
¼ cup water

¾ cup shredded cheddar, Swiss, or your
   preferred cheese

1. In a medium saucepan, combine the cream cheese, heavy cream, and water. Cook over low heat until the cream cheese has melted.

2. Add the shredded cheese ¼ cup at a time, stirring until it has melted before adding more. When the cheese has fully melted, about 5 minutes total, and the sauce has formed, remove from the heat. Let cool, or serve warm.

■ PREP TIP: Once fully cooled, this sauce can be stored in the refrigerator for up to 3 days. Simply reheat in the microwave, and stir thoroughly.

PER SERVING (¼ CUP): Calories: 272; Fat: 26g; Protein: 8g; Total carbs: 2g; Fiber: 0g; Net carbs: 2g

MACROS: Fat: 86%; Protein: 11%; Carbs: 3%

Sun-Dried Tomato Cream Cheese

MAKES: about 1½ cups | **PREP TIME:** 10 minutes

Sun-dried tomatoes are my favorite kind of tomato. They have a uniquely perfect balance of sweet and tangy. This recipe pairs them with cream cheese for a full flavor explosion. You can use this as a spread for keto bread or bagels or even as a dip for crunchy vegetables.

1 (8-ounce) package full-fat cream cheese, at room temperature
½ cup julienne-cut oil-packed sun-dried tomatoes

1. Using an electric hand mixer, in a medium bowl blend the cream cheese and sun-dried tomatoes on medium speed for 2 minutes, or until the cream cheese is smooth.

2. Serve, or store in an airtight container in the refrigerator for up to 10 days.

■ **INGREDIENT TIP:** If you can't find sun-dried tomatoes packed in oil, you can purchase the dry ones and use a tablespoon of olive oil.

PER SERVING (¼ CUP): Calories: 141; Fat: 13g; Protein: 3g; Total carbs: 4g; Fiber: 1g; Net carbs: 3g

MACROS: Fat: 82%; Protein: 8%; Carbs: 10%

Cowboy Chili-Cheese Dip

NUT-FREE

MAKES: about 3 cups | **PREP TIME:** 15 minutes | **COOK TIME:** 20 minutes

Texas has great chili and great queso. Pair the two together and be prepared for a complete flavor party. Deep hearty chili marries with a creamy delicious cheese sauce, leaving an absolutely unforgettable combination. Serve this with your favorite keto chip or cracker replacement, and give your guests a taste of Texas!

1 pound ground beef
⅓ cup diced onion
3 garlic cloves, minced
1½ teaspoons kosher salt, divided, plus more as needed
2 tablespoons ancho chili powder
½ teaspoon ground cumin
1½ cups water
2 tablespoons tomato paste

2 ounces cream cheese, at room temperature
1¾ cups shredded medium cheddar cheese, divided
Sour cream, for garnish
Diced avocado, for garnish
Chopped tomato, for garnish
Black olives, for garnish
Chopped fresh cilantro or parsley, for garnish

1. In a large sauté pan or skillet, combine the beef, onion, garlic, and ½ teaspoon of salt. Cook over medium heat for 5 to 7 minutes, or until the beef is no longer pink and begins to caramelize and the onion is tender.

2. Add the chili powder and cumin. Cook for 1 minute.

3. Stir in the water, tomato paste, and remaining 1 teaspoon of salt. Simmer for 2 to 3 minutes, or until the mixture thickens some. Taste the chili, and add more salt as needed.

4. Stir in the cream cheese until melted. Remove from the heat. Add 1½ cups of cheddar cheese, and stir until fully incorporated.

5. Pour the chili mixture into a small casserole dish, and cover until ready to serve.

6. When ready to serve, preheat the oven to 400°F.

7. Top the chili mixture with the remaining ¼ cup of cheddar cheese. Transfer the casserole dish to the oven, and bake for 7 to 10 minutes, or until the dip is bubbly. Remove from the oven.

8. Garnish with the sour cream, avocado, tomato, olives, and cilantro as desired for serving.

PER SERVING (¼ CUP): Calories: 173; Fat: 12g; Protein: 15g; Total carbs: 2g; Fiber: 1g; Net carbs: 1g

MACROS: Fat: 60%; Protein: 35%; Carbs: 5%

Crab and Artichoke Dip

NUT-FREE

MAKES: 2 cups | **PREP TIME:** 10 minutes | **COOK TIME:** 25 minutes

The paprika and Old Bay seasoning in this dip truly give it a distinct flavor profile. They pair well with slightly tart cream cheese and the mild yet nutty flavor of artichoke. Once you combine all of these ingredients with fresh crab, you surely have a winner. Served hot, this dip will keep your guests coming back to the table for more.

2 tablespoons extra-virgin olive oil
½ small onion, chopped
½ cup chopped artichoke hearts
1 cup frozen spinach, thawed and
    drained
2 garlic cloves, minced
8 ounces full-fat cream cheese, at room
    temperature

4 ounces crabmeat
1 teaspoon smoked paprika
1 teaspoon kosher salt, or Old Bay
    seasoning
½ to 1 teaspoon red pepper flakes
¼ cup mayonnaise
¼ cup freshly shredded Parmesan
    cheese

1. Preheat the oven to 375°F.

2. In a medium skillet, heat the oil over medium heat.

3. Add the onion, and sauté for 6 minutes, or until tender.

4. Add the artichoke hearts and spinach. Sauté for 4 to 5 minutes, or until the vegetables are tender and any water has evaporated.

5. Add the garlic and cream cheese. Cook, stirring constantly, for 3 to 4 minutes, or until the cheese is melted and creamy.

6. Reduce the heat to low. Stir in the crabmeat, paprika, salt, and red pepper flakes. Remove from the heat.

7. Add the mayonnaise and stir until creamy and well combined. Transfer to an 8-inch square glass baking dish, spreading the mixture out evenly.

8. Top with the Parmesan cheese.

9. Transfer the baking dish to the oven, and bake for 8 to 10 minutes, or until the cheese is melted and lightly browned. Remove from the oven. Serve warm.

■ **INGREDIENT TIP:** If you'd like to leave out the crab, simply increase the amount of spinach by ½ cup. This will give you a flavorful spinach-artichoke dip.

PER SERVING (⅓ CUP): Calories: 288; Fat: 26g; Protein: 9g; Total carbs: 6g; Fiber: 2g; Net carbs: 4g

MACROS: Fat: 80%; Protein: 13%; Carbs: 7%

Queso Blanco Dip

NUT-FREE

SERVES: 8 | **PREP TIME:** 5 minutes | **COOK TIME:** 10 minutes

"Queso blanco" literally translates to "white cheese." It's a soft cheese popular in Mexican and Latin dishes. This recipe can be made with actual queso blanco or with white cheddar. It is best paired with your favorite keto chip or cracker. The green chiles amp up the flavor, and the cream cheese intensifies the creaminess of this dip.

½ cup heavy cream

3 ounces cream cheese

1 cup shredded Monterey Jack cheese

1 cup shredded queso blanco or other sharp white cheddar cheese

1 (4½-ounce) can diced green chiles, drained

½ teaspoon freshly ground black pepper

½ teaspoon ground cumin

1. In a small saucepan, melt together the heavy cream and cream cheese over medium heat, whisking until totally melted.

2. Stir in the Monterey Jack cheese, queso blanco, and green chiles. Remove from the heat.

3. Add the pepper and cumin. Stir well, and serve.

■ **VARIATION TIP:** Adding chopped jalapeños will introduce a little heat that pairs perfectly with the tanginess of the green chiles.

PER SERVING (2 TABLESPOONS): Calories: 193; Fat: 17g; Protein: 8g; Total carbs: 3g; Fiber: 0g; Net carbs: 3g

MACROS: Fat: 78%; Protein: 16%; Carbs: 6%

Guacamole

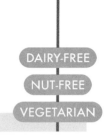

DAIRY-FREE

NUT-FREE

VEGETARIAN

Avocados are a huge staple in the keto diet. They are delicious, creamy, and packed with healthy fats. There are many variations of guacamole recipes, each with their own little twist. This dip is a classic recipe that is sure to please everyone in attendance. Feel free to throw in some chopped jalapeños for a spicy kick!

2 ripe avocados, peeled, pitted, and
   chopped
½ red onion, finely chopped
Juice of 1 lime
1 tablespoon egg white protein powder

2 teaspoons chopped fresh cilantro
1 teaspoon red pepper flakes
1 teaspoon minced garlic
Sea salt
Freshly ground black pepper

1. In a medium bowl, mash together the avocados, onion, lime juice, protein powder, cilantro, red pepper flakes, and garlic until mixed to your desired consistency.

2. Season with salt and pepper, and top with additional chopped onion and cilantro as you like. Transfer to a container. Cover, and refrigerate for up to 2 days.

PER SERVING (¼ CUP): Calories: 88; Fat: 7g; Protein: 2g; Total carbs: 6g; Fiber: 4g; Net carbs: 2g

MACROS: Fat: 70%; Protein: 8%; Carbs: 22%

Quick and Easy Ranch Dip

SERVES: 12 | **PREP TIME:** 10 minutes, plus 4 hours to chill

Ranch dip is easily a favorite across many households. This recipe lets you experience all the classic flavors of ranch without any extra additives. You can alter this recipe to make it to your liking. For example, add some red pepper flakes to turn it into a spicy ranch dip. It's perfect to eat with crunchy vegetables and is also great on sandwiches and salads.

1 cup heavy cream

1 tablespoon distilled white vinegar

¾ cup plain, full-fat Greek yogurt

1 teaspoon freshly squeezed lemon juice

2 teaspoons dried parsley

1 teaspoon dried dill

1 teaspoon dried chives

½ teaspoon garlic powder

½ teaspoon onion powder

½ teaspoon kosher salt

¼ teaspoon freshly ground black pepper

1. In a quart-size canning jar, combine the cream and vinegar. Set aside for 5 minutes.

2. Add the yogurt and lemon juice. Stir or shake the jar well.

3. Add the parsley, dill, chives, garlic powder, onion powder, salt, and pepper. Stir until thoroughly mixed. Put the lid on the jar, and refrigerate for 4 hours or overnight for the flavors to combine.

PER SERVING (2 TABLESPOONS): Calories: 79; Fat: 8g; Protein: 1g; Total carbs: 2g; Fiber: 0g; Net carbs: 2g

MACROS: Fat: 87%; Protein: 6%; Carbs: 7%

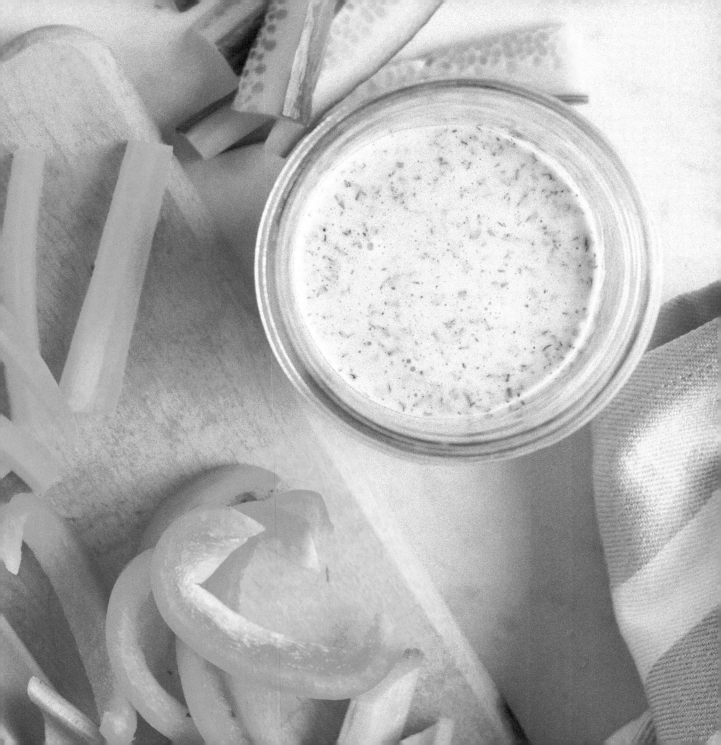

Herby Yogurt Dip

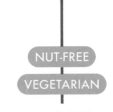

MAKES: about 1½ cups | **PREP TIME:** 10 minutes

This fresh, herb-filled, yogurt-based dip can take on a variety of roles. You can use it with grilled meats for a slight Mediterranean flair. You can place it in the middle of a spread of crunchy vegetables. You could even serve this cool creamy dip with keto-friendly Onion-Garlic Pita-Style Bread (page 78).

1 cup plain, whole-milk Greek yogurt
¼ cup extra-virgin olive oil
¼ cup chopped fresh parsley
1 tablespoon freshly squeezed lemon juice
1 tablespoon chopped fresh dill, or 1 teaspoon dried

1 tablespoon chopped fresh oregano, or 1 teaspoon dried
1 teaspoon garlic powder
1 teaspoon kosher salt
½ teaspoon freshly ground black pepper
Assorted raw vegetables, for serving

1. In a medium bowl, combine the yogurt, oil, parsley, lemon juice, dill, oregano, garlic powder, salt, and pepper. Whisk well until smooth and creamy.

2. Serve the dip with raw vegetables. Store in an airtight container in the refrigerator for up to 4 days.

■ **PREP TIP:** Add any additional light-tasting oil of your choice to help thin out the dip.

PER SERVING (¼ CUP): Calories: 109; Fat: 10g; Protein: 2g; Total carbs: 3g; Fiber: 0g; Net carbs: 3g

MACROS: Fat: 84%; Protein: 6%; Carbs: 10%

Creamy Spinach Dip

NUT-FREE

Spinach dip is another fan favorite. It's ooey, gooey, and cheesy, and this version includes ranch seasoning for a special twist. Because spinach dip tends to lean towards the salty side, it is best served with vegetables. However, feel free to serve this with bread or crackers as well.

Nonstick cooking spray

1 (10-ounce) package frozen spinach, thawed, drained, and squeezed dry

8 ounces cream cheese

8 ounces sour cream

2 tablespoons ranch seasoning

½ cup grated Parmesan cheese

1. Preheat the oven to 350°F. Spray an 8-by-8-inch baking dish with nonstick cooking spray.

2. In a small bowl, combine the spinach, cream cheese, and sour cream until well blended. Stir in the ranch seasoning.

3. Spread the mixture in the prepared baking dish. Sprinkle with the Parmesan cheese.

4. Transfer the baking dish to the oven, and bake for 20 minutes, or until the cheese has melted. Remove from the oven.

■ **PREP TIP:** Ensure the spinach is thoroughly dried so that it no longer releases water during the heating process.

PER SERVING: Calories: 275; Fat: 25g; Protein: 7g; Total carbs: 6g; Fiber: 2g; Net carbs: 4g

MACROS: Fat: 81%; Protein: 10%; Carbs: 9%

Smoky "Hummus" and Veggies

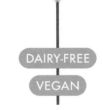

DAIRY-FREE

VEGAN

SERVES: 6 | **PREP TIME:** 15 minutes | **COOK TIME:** 20 minutes, plus 30 minutes to cool and chill

Unlike a standard hummus recipe, this version gets its creaminess from tahini and cauliflower rather than chickpeas, which are much higher in carbs. The combination of tahini and olive oil provide a good amount of healthy fats to fill you up quickly. Serve this delicious dip with fresh vegetables, such as celery and cucumbers.

Nonstick coconut oil cooking spray
1 head cauliflower, cut into florets
¼ cup tahini
¼ cup cold-pressed olive oil, plus more for drizzling
Juice of 1 lemon
1 tablespoon ground paprika

1 teaspoon sea salt
¼ cup chopped fresh parsley
2 tablespoons pine nuts (optional)
Flaxseed crackers, for serving
Sliced cucumbers, for serving
Celery pieces, for serving

1. Preheat the oven to 400°F. Grease a sheet pan with cooking spray.

2. Spread the cauliflower out on the prepared sheet pan.

3. Transfer the sheet pan to the oven, and bake for 20 minutes. Remove from the oven. Let cool for 10 minutes.

4. Put the cauliflower, tahini, oil, lemon juice, paprika, and salt in a food processor or high-powered blender. Blend on high speed until a fluffy, creamy texture is achieved. If the mixture seems too thick, slowly add a few tablespoons of water until smooth. Scoop into an airtight container, and refrigerate for about 20 minutes. Transfer to a serving bowl.

5. Drizzle with olive oil.

6. Garnish with the parsley and pine nuts (if using).

7. Serve the hummus with your favorite flaxseed crackers and sliced cucumbers and celery.

PER SERVING: Calories: 179; Fat: 15g; Protein: 5g; Total carbs: 10g; Fiber: 4g; Net carbs: 6g

MACROS: Fat: 72%; Protein: 8%; Carbs: 20%

Buffalo Chicken Dip

NUT-FREE

Buffalo might as well be synonymous with game day. You're bound to find some variation of Buffalo on any party table or appetizer menu. This dip is creamy, cheesy, and spicy. What more could anyone ask for? It features multiple types of cheese and cayenne for that famous Buffalo kick. It packs a punch and will surely be the center of attention.

8 tablespoons (1 stick) butter
1 teaspoon minced garlic
4 boneless chicken thighs
¼ cup sour cream
¼ teaspoon kosher salt
¼ teaspoon freshly ground black pepper
¼ teaspoon cayenne

¼ teaspoon paprika
8 ounces cream cheese, at room temperature
½ cup hot sauce, plus more as needed
½ cup ranch dressing
1 cup shredded mozzarella cheese
½ cup shredded cheddar cheese

1. Preheat the oven to 450°F.

2. Heat a large skillet over medium-high heat. Toss in the butter, and melt it.

3. Add the garlic and chicken. Cook for 3 minutes.

4. Reduce the heat to medium. Turn the chicken so it cooks on all sides for 12 to 15 minutes total, or until a meat thermometer reads 165°F. Remove from the heat. Transfer the chicken to a large bowl. Let cool, then shred into bite-size pieces.

5. Add the sour cream, salt, pepper, cayenne, and paprika. Mix well.

6. Spread the cream cheese over the bottom and up the sides of a 9-inch square baking pan, coating evenly.

7. Pour the chicken mixture over the cream cheese layer.

8. Drizzle the hot sauce and ranch dressing over the chicken mixture, distributing it evenly.

9. Top with the mozzarella cheese and cheddar cheese. Using a butter knife, swirl the ingredients together in the pan.

10. Transfer the pan to the oven, and bake for 15 minutes, or until the top layer is browned and bubbling. Remove from the oven. Let cool for 5 minutes before serving.

■ INGREDIENT TIP: This dish can be made with chicken breasts instead of chicken thighs.

PER SERVING: Calories: 417; Fat: 37g; Protein: 18g; Total carbs: 3g; Fiber: 0g; Net carbs: 3g

MACROS: Fat: 79%; Protein: 18%; Carbs: 3%

Cheesy Shrimp Spread

NUT-FREE

MAKES: 1½ cups | **PREP TIME:** 10 minutes

Savory shrimp is added to cream cheese and mayonnaise to form a different yet delicious spread. You can increase the amount of red pepper flakes to wake up your taste buds even more. This dip is best with cool crunchy veggies since it already packs a ton of flavor.

6 ounces cream cheese, softened
¼ cup mayonnaise
6 ounces cooked shrimp, chopped
1 tablespoon freshly squeezed lemon
    juice

1 tablespoon chopped scallions, both
    white and green parts
1 teaspoon chopped fresh dill
Pinch red pepper flakes
Sea salt
Freshly ground black pepper

1. Put the cream cheese, mayonnaise, shrimp, lemon juice, scallions, dill, and red pepper flakes in a food processor. Pulse until the spread is thick and well blended.

2. Season with salt and pepper. Refrigerate in a sealed container for up to 4 days.

PER SERVING (3 TABLESPOONS): Calories: 142; Fat: 13g; Protein: 6g; Total carbs: 1g; Fiber: 0g; Net carbs: 1g

MACROS: Fat: 78%; Protein: 18%; Carbs: 4%

Pimento Cheese

NUT-FREE

SERVES: 4 to 6 | **PREP TIME:** 5 minutes

Pimentos are tiny peppers that are big on sweet but not on heat. You can find pimento cheese in the deli section of most grocery stores. However, homemade is much better. This tangy spread is perfect for placing on top of bread, stirring into deviled egg mixtures (try it as a variation of the Bacon–Blue Cheese Deviled Eggs on page 22), or even devouring with crunchy celery sticks.

4 ounces full-fat cream cheese, at room temperature

¼ cup mayonnaise

2 tablespoons pimentos, drained and chopped

½ teaspoon kosher salt

¼ to ½ teaspoon cayenne, or red pepper flakes

1 cup freshly shredded extra-sharp cheddar cheese

1. In a medium bowl, combine the cream cheese, mayonnaise, pimentos, salt, and cayenne. Whisk until well combined, smooth, and creamy.

2. Stir in the cheddar cheese, and mix until well incorporated. Serve chilled, or cover and store in the refrigerator for up to 4 days.

■ **INGREDIENT TIP:** Use leftover pimentos in salads or inside a deviled egg mixture for a delicious, tangy surprise.

PER SERVING (2 TABLESPOONS): Calories: 307; Fat: 29g; Protein: 9g; Total carbs: 2g; Fiber: 0g; Net carbs: 2g

MACROS: Fat: 86%; Protein: 11%; Carbs: 3%

Baba Ghanoush

SERVES: 8 | **PREP TIME:** 15 minutes | **COOK TIME:** 45 minutes to 1 hour

Baba ghanoush is a popular Mediterranean-style dip. It has an eggplant base and often reminds people of hummus. This can be served with warm Onion-Garlic Pita-Style Bread (page 78), cucumbers, or celery. I love it with roasted bell peppers.

1 medium eggplant (1 to 1½ pounds)
¼ cup tahini
2 tablespoons freshly squeezed lemon juice
2 tablespoons olive oil, plus more for drizzling

1 teaspoon garlic powder
½ teaspoon kosher salt
Seeds from ¼ pomegranate
Chopped fresh parsley, for garnish

1. Preheat the oven to 350°F. Place aluminum foil on the middle rack.

2. Place the eggplant on the foil, and bake for 45 minutes to 1 hour, or until the eggplant is fork tender and the skin is very wrinkly. Remove from the oven. Let cool.

3. Once cool enough to handle, cut the eggplant lengthwise. Scoop out the flesh, and discard the skin and any liquid. Transfer it to a food processor or blender.

4. Add the tahini, lemon juice, oil, garlic powder, and salt. Blend for 2 minutes, or into a paste. Transfer to a serving bowl or plate.

5. Garnish with the pomegranate seeds, or arils, and parsley. Drizzle with olive oil.

■ **VARIATION TIP:** Add a couple teaspoons crushed red pepper flakes to give your guests a spicy version of this dip.

PER SERVING (2 TABLESPOONS): Per Serving: Calories: 99; Fat: 8g; Protein: 2g; Total carbs: 7g; Fiber: 3g; Net carbs: 4g

---

MACROS: Fat: 66%; Protein: 7%; Carbs: 27%

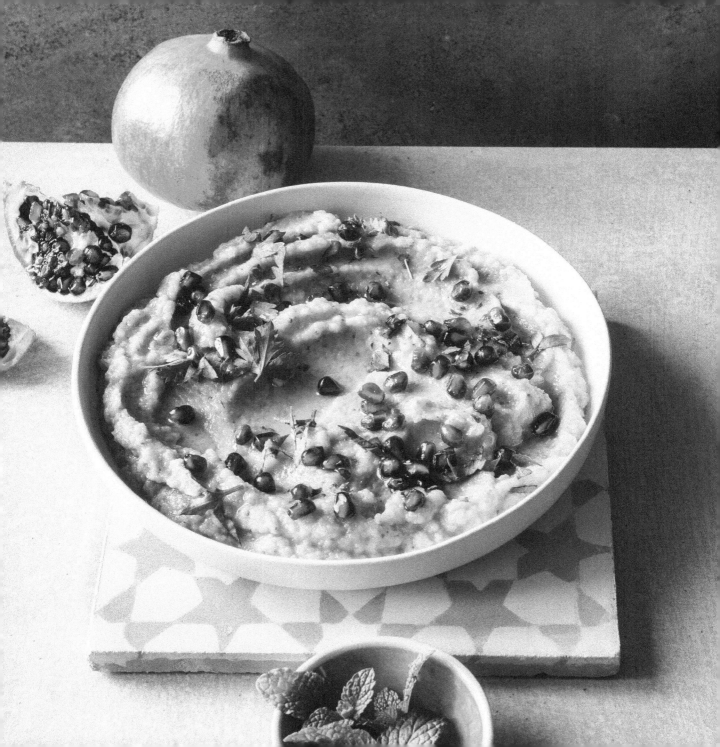

Olive Pâté

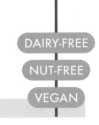

DAIRY-FREE

NUT-FREE

VEGAN

SERVES: 6 | **PREP TIME:** 10 minutes

This pâté, also known as a tapenade, is an olive overload. It's a simple recipe to follow, and it's full of healthy fats that keep you going. Traditionally, it is served on top of tiny pieces of toast. Feel free to whip out your favorite keto bread replacement and toast it for a delicious treat.

1 cup pitted green olives
1 cup pitted black olives
¼ cup cold-pressed olive oil

1 teaspoon freshly ground black pepper
2 thyme sprigs, leaves only
Crackers, for serving

1. Put the green olives, black olives, oil, pepper, and thyme in a food processor. Pulse until the mixture is thick and chunky. Transfer to a small serving bowl.

2. Serve the pâté with crackers.

■ **VARIATION TIP:** Would you like to try this out as a sauce? Add extra olive oil and lemon juice to create a savory sauce for use with noodles or on top of protein.

PER SERVING: Calories: 131; Fat: 14g; Protein: 0g; Total carbs: 3g; Fiber: 1g; Net carbs: 2g

MACROS: Fat: 91%; Protein: 1%; Carbs: 8%

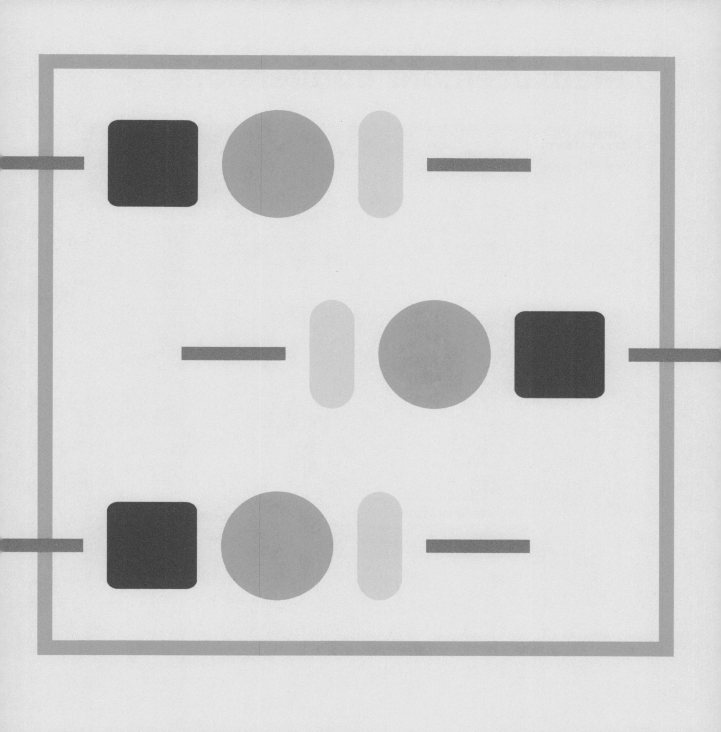

Measurement Conversions

VOLUME EQUIVALENTS	U.S. STANDARD	U.S. STANDARD (OUNCES)	METRIC (APPROXIMATE)
LIQUID	2 tablespoons	1 fl. oz.	30 mL
	¼ cup	2 fl. oz.	60 mL
	½ cup	4 fl. oz.	120 mL
	1 cup	8 fl. oz.	240 mL
	1½ cups	12 fl. oz.	355 mL
	2 cups or 1 pint	16 fl. oz.	475 mL
	4 cups or 1 quart	32 fl. oz.	1 L
	1 gallon	128 fl. oz.	4 L
DRY	⅛ teaspoon	–	0.5 mL
	¼ teaspoon	–	1 mL
	½ teaspoon	–	2 mL
	¾ teaspoon	–	4 mL
	1 teaspoon	–	5 mL
	1 tablespoon	–	15 mL
	¼ cup	–	59 mL
	⅓ cup	–	79 mL
	½ cup	–	118 mL
	⅔ cup	–	156 mL
	¾ cup	–	177 mL
	1 cup	–	235 mL
	2 cups or 1 pint	–	475 mL
	3 cups	–	700 mL
	4 cups or 1 quart	–	1 L
	½ gallon	–	2 L
	1 gallon	–	4 L

OVEN TEMPERATURES

FAHRENHEIT	CELSIUS (APPROXIMATE)
250°F	120°C
300°F	150°C
325°F	165°C
350°F	180°C
375°F	190°C
400°F	200°C
425°F	220°C
450°F	230°C

WEIGHT EQUIVALENTS

U.S. STANDARD	METRIC (APPROXIMATE)
½ ounce	15 g
1 ounce	30 g
2 ounces	60 g
4 ounces	115 g
8 ounces	225 g
12 ounces	340 g
16 ounces or 1 pound	455 g

Index

Acknowledgments

I'd first like to thank my parents for continuously pushing me to be the best and healthiest version of myself. Having an overweight child isn't easy, but they did their best to instill confidence in me and, at the same time, encourage me to live a healthier lifestyle. I remember my mom joining various exercise programs with me, even though she had no weight to lose!

I would also like to thank my husband. I recently had my first child, and trying to lose weight postpartum has not been easy—he has been nothing but supportive. Without all of these people, I would not have had the drive to continue on in what seems like a never-ending health and fitness journey.

About the Author

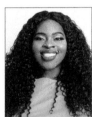 Hi, I'm Damilola Apata! After earning my bachelor's and master's degrees in accounting from Baylor University, I quickly realized I had no interest whatsoever in that field. Although I currently work in insurance and real estate, I like to spend my free time researching health and nutrition, creating delicious recipes, and spending time with my son and husband.

My favorite place in the house is the kitchen. I love that there are so many ways to create tasty meals and stay aligned with your nutritional goals. I have been following a low-carb lifestyle since 2017. In that time I've learned so many tips, tricks, and techniques to continue enjoying my favorite foods, and I love to share them with others.